The Death of Medicine

Piso Mojado

Foreword

This book is based upon actual events and upon the actions of famous surgeons. The Hungarian doctor who is the subject of this novel is often called by historians, "The savior of women" or "The savior of mothers".

This story is a drama that in many ways has not yet concluded. At first thought it would seem that we citizens of the twenty-first century are too wise as to allow the dominance of petty selfishness, hubris, and prejudices to trump the survival of so many innocent victims, as happened in Doctor Semmelweis's time. We have grown too much as a race to ever slide back into the unhappiness and darkness of the mid-nineteenth century, haven't we? We would quickly unite to ostracize any person, no matter what his or her wealth or position, whose lies or subterfuge was exposed as jeopardizing any innocent soul under his or her governance, wouldn't we? We would mock and shun any group or philosophy that placed short-term benefits for the few above a core set of common moral principles, wouldn't we?

Whether Moderate, Liberal, Conservative, wealthy or poor, northern or southern, eastern or western, young or old, Catholic or Protestant or Jewish or Other, there are certain values that we have learned by sad experience must be placed above monetary profit and religious and sectarian prejudice. Haven't we? We have learned too much from the the devastating world wars that mid-nineteenth century Europe spawned by not solving its own era's critical social, political, and economic issues not to have the courage to confront senseless ambition. Haven't we?

And yet, in these last few days of 2012, as I recheck this account of the life of Doctor Ignaz Semmelweis, I have heard on the news that medical instruments used in operations were found by reporters to be badly contaminated. On another network I heard an official of the federal agency responsible for the oversight of medical procedures explain to a reporter that contaminated operating rooms are not much of a problem. A minute later I heard one of the victims describe the agonizing months since he was infected in the hospital. There but for fortune go you or I. One small twist of destiny and we are in the shoes of that badly wounded victim thrust into the medicine of Doctor Semmelweis's era.

Do you sometimes have the nagging thought, then, reader, that the simple ideal of being responsible and ethical is not quite the situation of our time, that less disciplined men and women may have come to power, full of demagoguery, hypocrisy, excessive pride, and clever dialogue, ready to sweep away every advance in sense and conscience that humanity has achieved? I have those suspicions, too. I see much in the attitudes, events, divisions, delusions, and incomprehensible errors of mid-nineteenth-century Europe that are reflected in our present idiocies. That is one reason I was bound to the story of Doctor Ignaz Semmelweis. We could not believe that the events in this book could ever have happened, so patently unnecessary are they, unless we ourselves could look up from the page to our television, newspaper, or internet and see nearly identical folly. This book could not have been written ten years ago. In a wiser time this novel would seem like not-very-believable science fiction.

Could medicine revert to its disastrous past? I don't know. I do think that we all need to appreciate the immense distance that science has traveled. I believe we need to remind ourselves and each other to be grateful for the medicine we now have. We need to rededicate ourselves to protecting that medicine from corruption, bad law, special interest, and political bombast.

Yes, we have antibiotics now, although there are warnings that soon antibiotics may not be effective in fighting disease. We have investigative reporters to shine a light on practices that might deprive the innocent of life, although there are many that resent this press freedom (if it interferes with their profits or religious and political prejudices). We have television and the internet, which quickly tell us what poison or pitfall to avoid if we want to survive. We are fortunate. We need to recall what we have gained so that we can preserve these advances. We need to remember the desperation of the past.

The women of mid-nineteenth century Europe had only Doctor Ignaz Semmelweis.

The life of Doctor Semmelweis, then, is a commentary on so much more than just one of the greatest medical mysteries of all time. It is about well-trained men, honored to this day, who still have medical procedures and instruments named after them. These geniuses saw the simple truth in front of them again and again and yet refused to believe it.

It is about what is now called the "Semmelweis reflex", an instinct to reject the clear truth if it is in opposition to well-established ignorance.

This book is about brilliant men, the most educated professors at the most prestigious medical institution in the world, placing their standing in the world above the sanctity of human life. It is also about the converse, one

2

flawed man keeping his convictions even when the greatest men of the era ridiculed him. It is about courage and dedication, and doubts and persistence in the face of them. Above all, it is about how much one man kept caring, over and over again.

I want to insist that Semmelweis has remade our world, preparing the way for the germ theory (how did we ever come to accept that some nefarious invisible creatures make us sick?) and easing the path for other pioneers like Louis Pasteur, who is often credited as offering scientific hypotheses for Semmelweis's startling successes.

Why is the name 'Ignaz Semmelweis' still so obscure? During my research for this book I read again and again how Semmelweis's personality was the reason that his truths could not be accepted, how in his final years he acted the mad man and repelled those who might otherwise have accepted his successes. I do not see the history of Semmelweis in that light at all. I have to wonder if this impression is only a leftover from the nineteenth century, a condemnation of the prophet himself as a rationalization for wasting so many lives in spite of Doctor Semmelweis's vision.

Whether Doctor Semmelweis let others speak for him, as he did most of his career, or raged at the medical establishment, as he did in his final years, clearly made not a whit of difference. No doctor could have failed to see that Doctor Semmelweis was accomplishing miracles everywhere he served. No doctor, let alone any citizen of ordinary status, could have not realized the truth of Semmelweis's observations. Who would risk themselves against the prevailing wisdom? No one. It was easier to demonize Semmelweis.

I visualize doctors who were too afraid of, or too invested in, the prevailing political climate in medical circles to promote his ideas. No one was to allow Semmelweis's revelations, no matter how gently he begged to be understood. It did not matter at all what tone of voice Semmelweis used to address the medical professors of his era. It did not matter how Semmelweis addressed his colleagues.

As to the righteous anger of Doctor Semmelweis, only a man who felt indifferent to suffering or who was fearful of a closer examination of his successes would have stayed mild-mannered. Doctor Semmelweis was possessed of neither of these inhibitions. Semmelweis's often-cited impolitic correspondence and writings occurred in the latter stages of his crusade, when he had given up on a soft-spoken presentation of his results. In addition, these lectures and "open letters" undoubtedly incited the worst kind of slanders about Semmelweis, some of which may have endured. Perhaps

3

his biographers should instead praise him for finally speaking out, and discount the claims of his mental deterioration as not provable. I will let my readers judge whether his rage was the result of syphilis and Alzheimer's Disease or the long-suppressed righteous anger of a dedicated savior of women.

I had never heard of Doctor Ignaz Semmelweis. Most people reading this introduction probably have not. Why is this supremely instructive story not told to everyone everywhere? The narrative of how he overcame the limitations of his training and the ignorance of his age is one of the most inspiring biographies of all time. Doctor Semmelweis could have lived a life of position and prestige, but his conscience would not allow him to abandon the poor mothers of the world. He transformed our world because he would not, he could not, surrender to age-old excuses. Rather, he chose to be the one-man opposition to ignorance and special interest. He considered the wisdom of the professors he had respected, often bowed to the superiority of those more experienced and established than he, and finally could only be satisfied by truly scientific explanation and solution.

Herein lies one of the most remarkable stories I have ever encountered. I hope I have done justice to a man who never received justice in his lifetime.

Childbed fever

Childbed fever, often called 'puerperal fever' in medical literature, is a bacterial infection which is most often contracted during childbirth or during examination of a woman's genital organs during dilation. During the era in which the events in this book occur, the mid-nineteenth-century, the concepts of bacteria, antiseptics, sterile techniques, and antibiotics were unknown. Childbed fever was often fatal since bacteria from material foreign to the mother's body would enter the blood stream and cause a type of blood poisoning, called 'puerperal sepsis' in medical literature. The bacteria introduced by methods which are not sterile can travel through the blood and create symptoms throughout the body.

Recently, major news networks have warned that there is a possibility that antibiotics are becoming ineffective, and, if that eventuality occurs, even small cuts can lead to fatal infections. "Childbed fever" is an antique word for this "blood poisoning" but the disease that is the center of focus of this book is still a modern concern.

In addition, several other surveys that have recently come my way complain that more than half of medical personnel do not disinfect their hands properly. It would be nice if we of the twenty-first century could feel superior to the attitudes of the great learned men of the mid-nineteenth-century, and to the arrogance, carelessness, and selfishness described in this book.

We're not there yet.

The Death of Medicine

Chapter One

The screams shot through the window of Vienna's First Clinic as if the woman were in the adjoining room, when in fact Herr Doctor Semmelweis could see that she was outside the clinic, nearly forty yards distant, and seemingly being dragged along the filthy street.

"Pay no attention to that woman," the doctor who was conducting Semmelweis's tour of the First Clinic advised.

"She looks to be in the late stage of pregnancy. She may even be in labor. Don't you think she may need our assistance?"

"She will be one of your first patients soon enough, Herr Doctor Semmelweis. But she doesn't want your help quite yet. She wants to give birth in the street."

"She wants to give birth in the street?"

"Yes, Herr Doctor. She does not want to give birth inside the First Clinic. She is terrified because she is giving birth today. Today she must come to this particular clinic. She would rather have given birth yesterday or tomorrow, when she would have been admitted to a different clinic. Now that she cannot hold the baby in, she will try to give birth in the street. I have seen this kind of behavior many times."

The woman was shrieking, "Please, no doctors. Don't let the doctors kill me, I beg of you."

"That woman thinks doctors are going to kill her? She's delusional. And aren't those orderlies from our clinic? Where are they dragging her?"

"Into the clinic, of course. They are following their orders. They are quite accustomed to women who are extremely reluctant to give birth in the First Clinic. They've seen many women try to give birth in the street. That way the women can claim they were intending to give birth here in the clinic, but they couldn't quite make it. If the baby is born on the way to the clinic, they still get free services for the infant. And the mother feels safer because no doctor has touched her."

"Please! Please, have mercy on me and my baby. I don't want to die! Please don't take me to the doctors. I don't want to die," the woman was screaming.

"Is she delirious?" Semmelweis asked. "Why would she want to give birth on the street? Why wouldn't she rather have us helping her give birth and then take her to a nice childbed with clean sheets? Doesn't the child get free services anyway if she gives birth inside the clinic?"

"Yes, of course. She gets the same benefits whether she gives birth in the clinic or in the street. But she knows that anyone giving birth today must go to the First Clinic," the other doctor answered. "She wants to go to the Second Clinic, where only midwives help women give birth. She would rather give birth in the street than be forced into the First Clinic. She would rather give birth in the street than allow doctors to touch her or her baby. She is afraid if doctors help her, she will soon die."

"She would rather give birth in a maternity clinic directed by midwives than one manned by trained physicians?"

"Yes, Herr Doctor. That woman prefers to be assisted by midwives, but she will not get her wish today."

"But surely the doctors and students here have much more knowledge than midwives. Some mothers-to-be prefer midwives? That's preposterous. Why would they?"

"Everywhere in Vienna the women of the impoverished classes believe that to give birth in the First Clinic is a death sentence. Because the First Clinic is run by doctors. They are told if a mother goes to the First Clinic, a doctor will assist her birth, and she will probably die."

"Of course doctors will help her to give birth. That's what doctors do. That is what doctors are trained to do. Doesn't she realize that?"

"If she gives birth a day later, she'll go to the Second Clinic of Vienna General Hospital. There are no doctors in the Second Clinic, but it is also a maternity clinic."

"What ridiculous superstitions these women hold. If she is ungrateful for the doctors here, she cannot be taken to the Second Clinic now? If she prefers midwives to doctors, then we should admit her to the Second Clinic."

"No. It is against the rules. Mothers in the last stages of giving birth go to the First Clinic or the Second Clinic on alternate days. There are no exceptions. Today that woman in the street must come here, to the doctors' clinic. She can scream all that she wants but she will not be admitted to the midwives' clinic."

"She would rather have a midwife assist her birth than a doctor? She has lost her senses. She should be happy that she is giving birth on a day when she will be cared for by trained doctors."

"Yes, Herr Doctor, you are quite right. Unfortunately, most women would rather go to the midwives' clinic. To that woman in the street this day today is a Death Day."

"A Death Day?"

"Yes, a Death Day. Because she will be cared for by doctors and not midwives. The poor women of Vienna call it a Death Day if they are to be taken to the maternity clinic run by physicians. The woman outside the window will try to plead her way into the Second Clinic. She will learn her begging will accomplish nothing. Eventually she will give up her resistance. The pain will become too intense. She will stop struggling and resign herself to her fate. She will realize she can only hope and believe that she will be one of the lucky mothers that will survive a doctor's care."

"One of the lucky mothers to survive a doctor? Such ignorance."

"My thoughts exactly, Herr Doctor Semmelweis. The director of the First Clinic, Herr Professor Klein, will be happy to hear of your opinion. I feel that I should inform you that we have only women of the lowest classes here, Herr Doctor. That is why these clinics were created long ago. For the lowest classes of Austria. The Church does not want these women killing their babies, so Church officials created clinics for the poorer classes. These types of maternity clinics are not even restricted to the Austrian Empire."

There were going to be many sad lessons that this Semmelweis was going to learn these first few weeks, Doctor Miller thought. He knew that Doctor Semmelweis had wished for a position that did not involve the care of poor mothers and mothers-to-be. Probably Semmelweiss also had heard that the maternity clinics were full of Liberal toadies. Doctor Miller, a fellow Conservative, sympathized with the difficulties that the new chief resident faced. Therefore, he had decided to help educate Semmelweis so he would not run afoul of their common political opponents. "Upper class women and bourgeois women give birth at home. They would never come to the First Clinic unless they were suddenly destitute. Our level of expertise in assisting births, nevertheless, is the best in the civilized world. We are all trained by the most skillful doctors in the world, even if many of them are foreign Liberals."

Doctor Miller remembered how shocking his initial weeks in the First Clinic had been. He warned his new chief resident, "You must resign yourself to the kind of women you will encounter every day, Herr Doctor. Disgusting specimens. Prostitutes. Women giving birth to bastards. Peasant women from the surround of Vienna.

"Like you, Herr Doctor Semmelweis, I would rather have been assigned a different specialty. Don't look surprised. Herr Professor Klein and I were told by Herr Professor von Rokitansky, who recommended you for this position, that you had wanted to be an internist. It does not matter. No one will care that this was not your choice of wards. We Conservatives all have sympathy for those so unfortunate as to be posted here." Herr Doctor Miller winked at Semmelweis. "However, as consolation, Herr Doctor, you will be entitled to dissect a lot of dead mothers and learn a great deal about human anatomy here. The great Liberals encourage it."

Entitled to dissect a lot of dead mothers? Semmelweis silently protested the callousness of Doctor Miller. Was this the attitude of everyone he was to supervise and teach? Already his mind was almost completely filled with the unexpected difficulties he was encountering on his first day as chief resident. "These women that are afraid of us--don't they realize that doctors are no longer like medieval barbers, that we are an equal part of Vienna General Hospital, that we are in the forefront of the revolution that's been happening in medicine in the last two decades?" How unappreciative these lower class women were.

"The women know only what they have been told again and again, that they will probably die if a doctor touches them."

"Where would they get an idea like that?"

"I don't know, Herr Doctor Semmelweis. These are not women of the decent classes, of course. They are from uneducated families. They are bound to harbor strange ideas. They all think that they are going to die if they are admitted to the First Clinic before they have given birth. That's incorrect, of course. I have often been told by Herr Doctor Breit, who previously held your post, that even in the worst months at least half of the women who are admitted to the First Clinic will survive childbirth and its aftermath."

Semmelweis thought that Doctor Miller was making some weird jest. "Are you saying that one-half of the women admitted here will die?"

"No, not at all, Herr Doctor Semmelweis. I am not saying that at all. I am stating that less than one-half of the women admitted to the First Clinic will succumb to a fatal fever. I was told this by your predecessor. Herr Doctor Breit kept track of the fatalities himself, and you will be similarly tasked. It is one of the duties of the chief resident. I am reasonably sure he told me that less than half of the mothers admitted to the First Clinic will die. I was also informed that the death rate seems to fluctuate wildly. And that many of the mothers are transported elsewhere to die, and are not counted in the mortality statistics. However, Herr Doctor Breit assured me that the First Clinic has never lost more than 40% of its patients in a month, although it's difficult to know what he did or did not include in those numbers."

Perhaps this Doctor Miller was leading some initiation ritual for the chief resident. Doctor Semmelweis decided to pretend that he believed this wild story told by his tour guide. He played along. "I find these numbers to be truly shocking. I assume there are only mothers-to-be admitted here. This is by reputation a specialty clinic, which indicates that childbirth assistance is the expertise here. The First Clinic does nothing but assist mothers-to-be in giving birth, am I right? Of what possible malady could so many women possibly be dying?"

"Well, childbed fever, of course. I surmise you have not had much training at maternity clinics. Women give birth, are taken from the room where they give birth, and are given a nice clean childbed in which to rest and recover, and yet many of them soon develop a mysterious high fever, which leads to their death.

Doctor Miller continued, "Yes, this is a maternity clinic, Herr Doctor. And just like any maternity clinic anywhere in Europe, these women drop like flies. I only tell you this as a friend and colleague so that you can be prepared for what you will witness. You'll get used to it. It's normal."

Was Doctor Miller trying to frighten him with these wildly exaggerated death rate statistics? "I have to assume then that the First Clinic is receiving the most unhealthy women in Vienna and the outer areas. Are most of these mothers extremely sick when they are admitted? Do they have terrible diseases before they give birth?"

"No. Almost all of them seem perfectly healthy. Does that surprise you?"

"Of course. The First Clinic is part of Vienna General Hospital. This is where the medical revolution for the entire world began, where Herr Professor von Rokitansky and Herr Doctor Skoda have changed the whole direction of medicine, where scientific medicine has been introduced. What could be a safer place for a healthy woman to give birth than this clinic? I find it hard to believe that so many women would be dying under the noses of Herr Professor von Rokitansky and Herr Doctor Skoda. I am of course not questioning the conclusions of my predecessor, Herr Doctor Breit. I only assume there has been some error in transcribing the numbers, or that perhaps you have heard them incorrectly. Herr Professor von Rokitansky and Herr Doctor Skoda would never allow such failure in this new era of scientific medicine. No matter what class to which the patients belonged."

Doctor Miller bristled when he heard the foreign Liberals, von Rokitansky and Skoda, being praised so lavishly by a fellow Conservative, although he himself sometimes grudgingly acknowledged the expertise of Skoda and von Rokitansky. "Yes, I heard you were a student of the great Liberals. Most of us were or are. I also will be graduated from the University of Vienna medical school next year. Baron von Rokitansky recommended you for the position of chief resident? Is that correct?"

"Yes, that's correct."

"That's quite a recommendation. A Liberal recommending you? No one is likely to question your credentials, if Baron von Rokitansky nominated you for chief resident. That should make these young doctors and medical students fall in line. So it's true that you're the choice of the Baron himself. That must be confining. But, of course, we all have to adjust to the Liberal dominance here. It probably will be better if you always remember that the Liberal Baron is a fanatic about his scientific medicine. He has all of us doing as many autopsies as we possibly can, so that we will all get very skilled at anatomy. You should cut up as many dead mothers as you possibly can. To make von Rokitansky and Skoda happy."

Doctor Semmelweis was becoming increasingly alarmed by the disrespectful attitude of Doctor Miller. He replied stiffly, "I myself also believe that the knowledge we gain from autopsies is what will make us-effective scientists. Autopsies give us in depth knowledge of the human body, and provide us with knowledge about disease. That expertise will lead us to cures for

11

disease."

"Yes, Herr Doctor. Even Herr Professor Klein would agree with you. However, if you don't mind my warning, you unfortunately are starting to sound like one of Baron von Rokitansky's toadies. I say that because too much praise of the Liberals will offend Herr Professor Klein. You do not want to be on the left side of the director of the First Clinic, Herr Doctor Semmelweis. Was your speech about the usefulness of autopsies a direct quote from the Great Liberal Herr Professor von Rokitansky?"

What curious afflictions of opinion this Doctor Miller possessed. "Yes, as a matter of fact. But you yourself said you've been doing a lot of autopsies? As part of the scientific revolution in medicine?"

"We all have to. The Baron loves autopsies. Autopsies and the 'scientific revolution' are synonymous to the Baron. He and Herr Doctor Skoda claim their predilection for autopsies began a bright new direction in medicine in 1823 here in Vienna General Hospital. Actually it was Herr Professor Klein who encouraged autopsies and who started the revolution. Because Herr Professor Klein is an Austrian Conservative, the Czech Liberals stole the credit for his innovations. You'll soon realize that's the way the medals get pinned here at Vienna General Hospital's First Clinic." Doctor Miller winked again. "To be fair, the Liberals now promote autopsies to the extreme, even more than Herr Professor Klein. They are diligent about ordering autopsies that the lawyers haven't requested. But within limits, of course. Within prudence. They say that since Baron von Rokitansky has come to Vienna General Hospital he has told every doctor in the First Clinic that they must perform autopsies only on the patients that have died."

"Only if a mother died? But why... Oh." A bad joke. "Yes, of course. But Baron von Rokitansky is correct."

"Don't let Herr Professor Klein hear you say that. Baron von Rokitansky is a Liberal and a Bavarian Czech. Our chief, Herr Professor Klein, is an Austrian and a Conservative. Anyway, if Baron von Rokitansky is correct about anything, it's an idea he stole from Herr Professor Klein."

"An Austrian and a Conservative? I don't understand. The whole scientific revolution in medicine is based on doctors having knowledge of human anatomy. I'm sure Herr Professor Klein must agree, does he not? What difference does politics make? The more autopsies, the more we can discover the similarities in the causes of a particular disease. For instance, when you autopsied the mothers who died here, did you discover an excess of the same one of the four humours in every case, or almost every case? Didn't the autopsies reveal some cause for these fevers that are killing the mothers?"

"No. We are administering to the damned here, Herr Doctor Semmelweis. We will not find God's curse inside an organ. Twenty years of autopsies have not cured the lower classes of their sins."

The cries of the woman outside were even louder. The orderlies were having some success moving the woman closer to the clinic, but she was still begging them not to take her before the doctors. "I don't want to be another dead body for the Baron. You want me for another autopsy. I know what goes on in there. The Baron needs another dead body. I know today is a Death Day. Please. Who will take care of my baby? Please. I don't want to die."

"She does not want to be another dead body for the Baron? She is speaking of Baron von Rokitansky?" Semmelweis asked.

"Yes, she is blessing your Liberal benefactor. These whores know everything that goes on in our hospital, Herr Doctor. They have heard the Baron has encouraged many more autopsies since he arrived many years ago with his new scientific methods."

"That is why the woman is afraid to give birth here? Because she has heard Baron von Rokitansky has greatly increased the number of autopsies? That is why she thinks the doctors are going to kill her?"

"Possibly. But mainly because it is a Death Day. That woman knows today is a Death Day. Mostly, the whore in the street doesn't want to be selected to come here because of the death rate in the First Clinic, not because of the autopsies. Or possibly she actually believes we encourage death here to burnish our reputation as healers."

Doctor Semmelweis understood that Doctor Miller enjoyed being cleverly sly, but he himself tried to ensure that his own tone did not encourage any further disrespect toward his own teachers or to the usefulness of scientific medicine. On the other hand, he did not want to make an enemy of Miller. He offered agreement to his tour guide, "Encourage death so we can have more bodies to examine? Nonsense, of course."

"Yes, nonsense. She is only an ignorant whore."

13

"But she is now one of our patients. She is now in our care, no matter what her beliefs. I am having difficulty understanding the situation. It bothers me that any mother-to-be would be afraid of scientific medicine. I'm sure our clinic gives the best care possible. I'm sure this woman understands that the danger that she imagines is exaggerated. After all, she knows that we are part of Vienna General Hospital. We are a beacon for the world. All Vienna must realize that we are giving mothers-to-be the most extraordinary care. Of course, if those numbers you told me about earlier were actually accurate...." Doctor Semmelweis rewarded his tour guide with an expression of extreme disgust and skepticism. Some doctors were spreading terrible lies about Vienna General Hospital's First Clinic for some twisted political reason.

"You should not say 'if', Herr Doctor, if you pardon my correction. Herr Professor Klein would be displeased to hear you have questioned the honesty of your predecessor's books."

Doctor Semmelweis did not want to caught in some trap set by a political fanatic. "I didn't mean that at all. I believe you told me the numbers fluctuate. You said the death rate statistics vary greatly." Was his new superior, Herr Professor Klein, also part of a plot to publicize fantastic death rate statistics to the general public? What possible reason could the director of the First Clinic have to destroy its reputation?

"That the numbers change each month should give you no consolation, Herr Doctor Semmelweis." Doctor Miller seemed to be enjoying the new chief resident's shock and discomfort. "I said that in some months the death rate is higher than in other months. They are, however, consistent within certain upper and lower limits."

"I see. I misunderstood." The First Clinic had had a bad month, so Doctor Miller was using a temporary aberration to slander the First Clinic and the scientific medical revolution. That is what Doctor Semmelweis heard between the lines. "But, anyway, what good does that woman think giving birth in the street will do? Why does she think she is going to have a better result if midwives help her deliver? Won't she die of fever just the same if she gives birth in the street? What good is giving birth in a filthy gutter? She will still get sick if her humours are unbalanced, no matter where she gives birth."

"No, to the contrary, surprisingly. Mothers who give birth in the street and then are placed in a childbed here rarely develop childbed fever. Somehow these mothers-to-be seem to know all this. It is as there is a spy that reads the chief resident's books."

"That can't be true! That doesn't make sense. Mothers that give birth in the street stay healthy? Something is terribly wrong with that observation. What kind of medical science is that? And it gives some credibility to the crazy idea that mothers develop a disease when a doctor helps them give birth."

"But it is true that mothers who give birth in the street--who are never examined by a doctor--rarely develop a fatal fever. Welcome to the depressing world of the First Clinic. Your predecessor as chief resident, Herr Doctor Breit, kept track of street births and the fatality rate of such births. You can ask Herr Director Klein about the registry of street births and the death rate, if you wish. I don't advise it. As I said earlier, the director of the clinic will not tolerate any skepticism about Doctor Breit's honesty. Herr Doctor Klein has been down that road many times too often. Anyway, you'll probably be recording the numbers yourself very soon."

"I was not questioning my predecessor's honesty. I only meant that it doesn't make sense that giving birth in the street is healthier than giving birth in a medical clinic."

Doctor Miller was amused by Doctor Semmelweis's stubbornness. "A lot of things make no sense here. Giving birth in the clinic run by midwives, for instance, is as healthy as giving birth in the street. That's why these women want to go to the other maternity clinic, the Second Clinic. These women know of the strange phenomenon--the curse of the First Clinic. I think these women have kept better statistics over the years than all of us, Herr Doctor Semmelweis. The poor women of Vienna are somehow very knowledgeable about which conditions favor their survival. Their medical intelligence for such an ignorant class is a remarkable phenomenon."

"Mothers giving birth in the street or attended by midwives have a better chance than those cared for by the best-trained surgeons in the world? That's outrageous. I'm sorry, Herr Doctor Miller, but I don't believe a word of what you are saying." Did this Austrian think he would frighten away the new chief resident so easily?

"None of us want to believe the facts, Herr Doctor. It is discouraging to every surgeon in the clinic. I prefer to think of us as the instruments of divine justice. As I told you, you're dealing with a different class of women than you are probably accustomed to, Herr Doctor. It's a strange situation. I have to believe the poor women of Vienna are damned."

15

"If the poor women of Vienna are damned, why aren't they cursed equally whether they enter the doctors' clinic or the midwives' clinic?"

"The ways of God's justice are a mystery to us mortals, Herr Doctor."

"So how much better could it be for a mother to give birth in the Second Clinic rather than here?"

"The monthly death rate in the midwives' clinic is usually one-third or less than that of the First Clinic. Last year we recorded 240 deaths due to childbed fever. The Second Clinic had a few more than sixty."

"One-third or less? 240 mothers died in the First Clinic? Ridiculous."

"That doesn't include those who were taken from the First Clinic to other parts of Vienna General Hospital in order to pass on. If we don't have enough room to allow the mothers to die here, they are taken from their childbed and transported elsewhere."

Doctor Semmelweis suppressed his horror at this news. He suspected that the numbers Doctor Miller was quoting were a mean invention and that he would learn after he had been chief resident a week or two that it was Doctor Miller who was strange and not the statistics. But what about the woman in the street? Her panic at being taken to see doctors was real. Was there some conspiracy of false death rate statistics, perhaps, that had been impressed on the women of Vienna to encourage them not to bother the doctors? What was going on here? The numbers that Miller was spouting could not possibly be real. So what was his purpose in verbalizing them? But Doctor Semmelweis must make no protest aloud. It was his first day as chief resident, and Doctor Miller had already warned him twice about any skepticism about the death rate statistics. There would be plenty of time in the coming days to sort out the questions he had about the woman trying to give birth in the street, about the numbers Doctor Miller had quoted, and about the alleged statistics kept by his predecessor, Doctor Breit.

Yet Doctor Semmelweis still felt compelled to be sure he had heard correctly the shocking difference in the number of deaths between the doctors' clinic and the midwives' clinic. "The Second Clinic recorded about 60 deaths last year, but our clinic had 240?"

"That is what I was told. Herr Doctor Semmelweis, a word to the wise. I am only telling you these things as a friend to the new chief resident. I can see by your expression that you are reluctant to accept the truth of the situation.

You will find out soon enough that everything that I am telling you is the reality. You must never speak of these statistics, however. Herr Professor Klein frowns on even the slightest mention of the midwives and the Second Clinic. Naturally, he does. He has severely reprimanded medical students for intimating that the midwives provide better care for the lower classes of mothers than we do. He would be apoplectic if he knew his new chief resident was also spreading that rumor."

"Yes, of course, Herr Doctor Miller." Semmelweis backtracked quickly. "I am sorry if I gave the impression that I was doubting the skill of the doctors and students here. I have, after all, been graduated myself From the University of Vienna Medical School."

"Yes, I know. The protege of Baron von Rokitansky and Doctor Skoda. Herr Professor Klein is impressed, especially since he has heard you are politically at odds with those Liberals."

"I am not political, Herr Doctor Miller."

Miller winked. "Yes, certainly. That is exactly the stance you should assume. And you must be very careful what you say about those Liberal gods. I don't blame you for your prudence. You are new. You are feeling out the strength of your opponents, as we all must. If you don't mind my giving you some advice, Herr Doctor, you will be wise to stay so careful and to confine your speech to medical matters. Also, you should be wary of crossing either of the great Liberals, Skoda or Rokitansky, if I might speak frankly as a friend. They have a lot of power and influence."

"I am only interested in becoming a better healer, as I am sure you are, Herr Doctor. Does the First Clinic administer to more mothers giving birth than the Second Clinic?"

"No, about the same."

"I am only trying to understand the situation. What are the differences between the two clinics?"

"Only that the First Clinic is run by doctors, Herr Doctor Semmelweis, and the Second Clinic is run by midwives."

"There must be some other difference."

"Herr Doctor, perhaps these questions should be posed to your supervisor,

Herr Professor Klein. But I advise against it. It would be better if you forgot the Second Clinic existed. No one speaks about the Second Clinic. It would not be good for anyone's career to be curious about the Second Clinic. We are doctors. The First Clinic and only the First Clinic is our concern. Now if there is some other part of this clinic you would like to see?"

"No, but I am naturally curious about the Second Clinic, of course."

"You are a very obstinate man, Herr Doctor Semmelweis. I have already strenuously advised you against such discussion. That subject would greatly displease the Herr Professor. We can go see him now, if you'd like. He is relieved to have another Conservative in the clinic. You will be pleased to learn that the director of the clinic is also a Conservative. But here in the First Clinic we are greatly outnumbered by the Liberals. The damn Bohemian Czechs are the number one force of opinion here. We needed an Austrian Conservative counter-balance like you, Herr Doctor Semmelweis."

Doctor Semmelweis began to protest. Miller winked and interrupted Semmelweis, "I could tell by your regal bearing, Herr Doctor Semmelweis, that you are one of us. Professor Klein was worried because his new assistant was pushed on him by von Rokitansky and Skoda, but I'll tell him you're a good old Austrian Conservative."

"I'm not political," Herr Doctor Semmelweis said icily. "And I am Hungarian."

The expression of horror on Miller's face told Semmelweis everything he didn't want to know about the doctor who would be under his supervision. Hungarian? The new chief resident was Hungarian? Herr Doctor Miller's attitude toward the new chief resident changed completely. The 'friend' did not say another word as he escorted Semmelweis to the office of the director of the First Clinic, Herr Doctor Klein.

Chapter Two

Doctor Semmelweis was left waiting over an hour outside the office of his new superior, Professor Johann Klein. The doctor who had been showing Semmelweis around his new home, the First Clinic,
had entered Professor Klein's office when they had first arrived, evidently to give the Professor a report about his new chief resident, but had departed only ten minutes previously.

Finally Semmelweis was permitted to see Professor Klein. The professor did not invite the newcomer to sit, and he himself remained standing as well.

"You're Hungarian, Herr Doctor Semmelweis?" the professor began stiffly. "I have just been informed of this. Is that true?"

"I was born in Hungary, Herr Professor."

"You're Hungarian then. I have to assume then that you are a Liberal."

Doctor Semmelweis was stunned at the assertion. "I am a doctor, Herr Professor. I have nothing at all to do with politics."

"You're Hungarian. I have never met a Hungarian who was not a Liberal. I have never even heard of a Hungarian who is not a Liberal. Unless you're one of those Hungarian Radicals that wants to get rid of the Emperor of Austria."

"I don't know how to answer you any further, Herr Professor. I am not political. Medicine is my life. My every waking minute is preoccupied with thoughts about medical matters. I do not have time for political matters."

"Young man, you are a Hungarian. There is no such thing as a Hungarian Conservative. I am no fool. You were recommended by Herr Baron von Rokitansky, a Czech Liberal, and Herr Doctor Skoda, another Czech Liberal. Now I know why. My worst fear was to have a chief resident who is disloyal and ungrateful to the Austrian Emperor."

"I am completely loyal to the Austrian Emperor. The Austrian Emperor is also the King of Hungary."

"That makes you a Liberal, then. Liberals want to keep the Emperor but force him to say 'please' and 'yes, of course' every time they have some petty demand. Radicals want to be free of the Austrian Emperor altogether. What do you think of Radicals, Semmelweis?"

"I am not political, Herr Professor. I do not know any Radicals."

"You were born in Hungary and you know of no Radicals?"

"Only by accounts in the newspapers, Herr Professor."

"Well, you do speak very good German, Semmelweis. You must have half of a good Austrian upbringing. You do understand that I must guard my clinic from an infection of Radicalism? But you say you are loyal to the Austrian Empire. You swear you are loyal to the Austrian Emperor?"

"Yes, I am completely loyal to the Austrian Emperor. And I learned to speak and write German at an early age."

"Well, better to have a Liberal than a Radical, I suppose. I thought I had heard you were an Austrian Conservative. I don't know how I got that idea. Perhaps Herr Baron von Rokitansky has deceived me. Are you a friend of the Baron's? Herr Professor von Rokitansky has been effusive in his praise."

"I could not be so presumptuous as to call myself a friend of the Baron. I was graduated from the University of Vienna Medical School. I was a student of Herr Baron von Rokitansky and Herr Doctor Skoda. I was trained in the methods of scientific medicine and in the techniques of the modern revolution in medicine that Vienna is teaching to the rest of the world. My only goal is to know the anatomy of the human body perfectly and to realize in which organ of the human body, which imbalance of the four humours, causes a particular disease. Autopsies are my politics, Herr Professor Klein. Human anatomy is my politics, Herr Professor. Finding ways to right the imbalance of humours, to correct the disequilibriums which cause human suffering--that is my only politics, Herr Professor Klein, and will be until the end of my life."

"A very good reply, Herr Doctor. A very good answer. I am impressed by your zeal. It almost borders on fanaticism to my ear. It is refreshing to hear someone so enthusiastic about medicine. Some doctors and students are becoming jaded. Perhaps your attitude will change them."

"Thank you, Herr Professor."

"I am equally dedicated to medicine. I am as committed to the Austrian revolution in medicine as your professors, if not more so. I am as eager to prevent Austrian medicine from sliding backward into a darkness of medieval ignorance and superstitions. That is why I do not want any Liberal political ideas in my clinic. I do not want such defeatism in my halls. I know your teachers well. Baron von Rokitansky is a Liberal. A Czech. A Bohemian. A Liberal. Doctor Skoda is a Liberal. A Czech. A Bohemian. A Liberal. I must always wonder if such men are grateful for the opportunity the Empire has granted them. I, Herr Doctor, am an Austrian, a Conservative who will always be loyal to the Habsburg Empire."

Semmelweis protested, "I am loyal to the Emperor. I am completely loyal to the Habsburg Empire. My teachers are also loyal, I assure you, Herr Professor. I have never heard one word against the Emperor at the University."

"Yes, yes. Of course you would not consider those Bohemian ideas to be anti-Austrian. You Liberals only want to 'reform' the Empire, even though your reforms will weaken the Empire, encourage people to challenge the authority of the Empire, and eventually destroy the Empire."

"Herr Professor, I am not political and do not understand that to which you refer. I assure you I have no wish for the Empire to be damaged in any way. I am a resident in the Empire. Why would I wish for such a calamity?"

Herr Professor Klein studied the face of his new chief resident. Had he sufficiently established his unchallengeable authority to this young doctor? Had he frightened this doctor enough? "I am the director of the First Clinic and I will not tolerate any weakling nonsense, Herr Doctor. Never forget that. I suspect that you are another Liberal, Semmelweis, and I am already drowning in Liberals. I must accept you as my new chief resident, but I'll be watching every move you make.

"You asked about the Second Clinic. Your first day as a chief resident at the first maternity clinic of the Vienna General Hospital and you try to undermine me by asking about the second maternity clinic, the midwives clinic?"

"No, Herr Professor, nothing of the sort. I was not trying to undermine you, and I would not try to weaken your authority. I wasn't even aware of the Second Clinic until Herr Doctor Miller mentioned it earlier." Semmelweis was now nearly positive that only minutes earlier Doctor Miller had been telling lies to Professor Klein. "Doctor Miller had told me that the Second Clinic has less than a third of the deaths of our clinic, Herr Professor. I was naturally curious as to why the Second Clinic should have fewer fatalities."

"Would you rather be a chief resident at the midwives' clinic, Herr Doctor?"

"No, of course not, Herr Professor."

"The First Clinic is for the training of doctors. The Second Clinic is for the training of midwives. The difference should be clear even for a Hungarian. You are to have nothing to do with the Second Clinic. Is that clear, Semmelweis?"

"Yes, Herr Professor."

"Has Herr Professor von Rokitansky and Herr Doctor Skoda recommended you so fiercely just so they could have someone who could use the Second Clinic to embarrass me? Are you some kind of Trojan Horse, Semmelweis?"

"No, Herr Professor, I did not mean to create that impression. I have just today heard of the Second Clinic."

"The midwives' clinic has always had a much better death rate than our clinic, Herr Doctor. Since it was created as a separate maternity clinic five years ago. No one knows why so many fewer mothers die in the Second Clinic. The matter has been thoroughly investigated, and no scientific reason has been found for the difference. No medical reason has been found for the difference in the death rate between the First and Second Clinics. Therefore, it should not be a matter for your concern."

"Yes, Herr Professor." Why was Professor Klein so sensitive about the subject of the Second Clinic? Was there truth to what Doctor Miller had been claiming earlier?

"Your duties will be to examine patients every morning in preparation for my rounds, to supervise difficult deliveries, to keep the statistics for the clinic, and to teach medical students. You will be training young doctors, not having midwives instruct you. Is that clear?"

"Yes, Herr Professor."

"Medicine is barbarous in Hungary, Semmelweis. You're in Austria now. Never forget that. Here we adhere to those scientific methods you have learned. You will also find that the study of medicine is much more complicated than you were led to believe at the University. You may not have realized what you were getting into."

"Yes, Herr Professor."

"I do not want to discourage you in your pursuit of excellence, but you should not think you will have all the answers on the first day. You must also confine yourself to the observation only of those jurisdictions that have been placed under your authority. That will be more than enough difficulty to occupy your every waking moment during the next two years. You will soon learn that trying to discover the innumerable causes of each sickness is nearly impossible.

"Even your benefactor, the Czech Liberal, has found how difficult it is to control the imbalance of the four humours, even with the new emphasis on anatomy we have instituted. Baron von Rokitansky has promised a revolution in medicine. So be it. But you should expect no quick progress in finding the causes of sickness, no matter how many post-mortems you conduct and supervise. But conduct and supervise, you will. You'll find much of the time in this hospital is spent doing autopsies. We've done thousands of autopsies here since the scientific revolution in medicine began."

"Thousands of autopsies?"

"I'm not exaggerating, Semmelweis. After all, it's been over two decades since we swept out all that ineffective philosophy, and decided that medicine was a matter of anatomy. It's been nearly twenty-five years since I became director of this clinic. I believe, like your professors, in the efficacy of studying human anatomy. I hope you do not have a sensitive nose."

"No, Herr Professor."

"We'll see. I was the one to begin the revolution in scientific medicine, not your benefactor, Herr Professor von Rokitansky. I began the increase in autopsies in 1823. Did you know that?"

"No, Herr Professor."

"And yet we still have the same diseases. Unfortunate. But I am expecting that July, 1846, will be a propitious month. Now that we have the student of the Liberal princes as our chief resident."

"I will do my best, Herr Professor."

"Semmelweis, I'm sure you are aware I was Professor of Obstetrics at the University of Salzburg and at your alma mater, the University of Vienna. I am an Austrian professor. I will take no position in the back of the lecture hall in deference to the Liberal gods. I am the arbiter of scientific medicine here in the First Clinic."

"Certainly, Herr Professor Klein."

"I received this position at the same time your benefactor was proclaiming the need for autopsies, and, like you, Semmelweis, I was convinced that a new approach to disease was the answer. I had the same enthusiasm then as you seem to have now. I thought I would turn the world of medicine on its head. I became director of this clinic because Herr Professor Johann Boer quit in 1822. Herr Professor Boer could not bear the deaths of so many mothers.

"I changed everything in this clinic. I revised the entire focus of medicine in the First Clinic. I knew that the more autopsies we did, the more we studied anatomy, the closer we would get to understanding why so many mothers were dying. I was sure I would create my own revolution. I would not end up like my predecessor, Herr Professor Boer, burned out and suicidal."

"Yes, Herr Professor."

"My medical methods are quite similar to those of your professors who started the 'scientific revolution in medicine'." Professor Klein pronounced the last four words sarcastically. "My political ideas are not."

"Yes, Herr Professor."

"When you familiarize yourself with the papers that your predecessor has left you, you may find that the death rate now is even much higher than when Herr Professor Boer left the clinic. That is quite a mystery. I have been here since 1822 and I have done everything correctly, Semmelweis. Yet my scientific revolution has changed nothing. I expect that you will have the same result. You should expect that you will have the same lack of success."

"Yes, Herr Professor."

"Many more mothers are dying now of childbed fever than when I arrived at the clinic or when the Baron began lecturing at the University. We all believed the more dead mothers we cut apart, the more mothers we would save. Nothing has changed; nothing will change. I agree that a knowledge of anatomy is of the utmost importance. But now I wonder if we must continue the autopsies at a torrid rate just to save face, even when much of the time there is no legal requirement for the postmortem.

"So much for the revolution in medicine, Semmelweis. I do not want us to retreat to the days to the days when medicine was a philosophy, not a science, but I also want my chief resident to accept matters as they currently exist. You will not change the situation in the First Clinic, Semmelweis. I can assure you of that. I know quite well that we cannot do more for the women of Vienna. All these years of expanded effort and no result. I am telling you this for your own good, Herr Doctor. I want you to begin your medical career on your strongest foot."

Doctor Semmelweis thought he would change the subject that had become so uncomfortable to him. He tried to flatter his new supervisor. "Yes, Herr Professor. I understand. I have recently studied your lectures, Herr Professor. How do you think I should concentrate the focus of the medical students?"

"Why on the imbalance of the four humours, of course. Make sure the students are bleeding their patients correctly. Make sure they are correctly measuring the amounts of the four humours during the autopsies. Your teachers may not have stressed the importance of careful postmortem techniques. It does no good to perform thousands of autopsies if doctors are not meticulous, if they are not Conservative in their methods. We practice only scientific medicine that pays attention to every detail. I will not tolerate sloppy work. I am telling you this for your own good, Herr Doctor. Do not earn a reputation for doing post-mortems too quickly and without complete thoroughness."

"Yes, of course, Herr Professor."

Professor Klein's expression seemed to soften a little. "Perhaps you will understand over time why I must resist the barbarian influence of the Liberals, Semmelweis. Perhaps you will learn to turn against your unnatural Hungarian tendencies. You will never be an Austrian, Semmelweis, but perhaps you can learn from us. You've undoubtedly been bent by the politics of Baron von Rokitansky and Herr Doctor Skoda. The Czech Liberals have wild political ideas, Semmelweis. On the other hand you do have a medical degree from the University of Vienna. You must have absorbed some

Austrian sense. Perhaps there is hope for you if you abandon the ignorance of the Czech Liberalism of your benefactors and the Hungarian Liberalism of your homeland."

"Yes, Herr Professor."

"You're father was a very wealthy Hungarian?"

"Yes, Herr Professor. He was famous for his wholesale spice business."

"Your mother is the daughter of the very famous Austrian vehicle builder?"

"Yes, Herr Professor, my father-in-law is famous for his horse-drawn coaches." Herr Professor Klein had known much more about Semmelweis than he had first revealed. His new supervisor, Semmelweis thought, seemed devious and a bit paranoid.

"That may help you some, Semmelweis. You should make this well-known. You're always going to be suspect, Semmelweis, being a Hungarian. You should subtly try to impress on others who your in-laws are. I'd like people to be aware that my chief resident is related by marriage to the famous Muller family."

"Yes, Herr Professor."

"Make sure that nothing comes out of your mouth that makes you seem like a Liberal. I do not want to be embarrassed by my chief resident."

"Yes, of course, Herr Professor."

"You will begin your rounds tomorrow morning. I will expect you to familiarize with the current cases, and then I will join on the following day. You are dismissed."

Chapter Three

The following morning, July 2nd, was not as terrible as Doctor Semmelweis had expected. He had begun examining patients in the First Clinic, introducing himself to the other doctors as the new assistant to Professor Klein. They were quite helpful in explaining the usual procedures in the First Clinic. He had expected a great deal of hostility because of his youth and because of the ambiguous welcome he had been given by Professor Klein and Doctor Miller, but he seemed to be regarded as a worthy colleague and supervisor by most doctors in the First Clinic. Yet Doctor Semmelweis was now acutely aware of his nationality, measuring his every word for anything that could possibly be interpreted as Liberalism.

On this second day Professor Klein was not to accompany Semmelweis on his rounds, so Semmelweis began to wander the clinic. Since this day was one in which all patients were directed to the Second Clinic, he had a good deal of free time to make observations about his new place of employment. Mainly, though, he wanted to avoid other people. He had been deeply stung by his meeting with Professor Klein.

In mid-afternoon a Doctor Eckhof took him aside. "I hope you excuse my boldness but you need to relax, Herr Doctor."

"Yes?"

"I can only assume that Professor Klein gave you the speech warning you about propagating any Liberal ideas."

Doctor Semmelweis was afraid to acknowledge the previous day's conversation with his superior. He feigned innocence. "The speech about Liberalism?"

"Almost every doctor here is a Liberal compared to Herr Professor Klein, Herr Doctor Semmelweis. It is a meaningless term in the context of the First Clinic. You don't have to be afraid. The panic is written all over your face. Herr Professor Klein tries to intimidate all of us. It's the initiation into the First Clinic. Herr Doctor, we're in the same terrible war now, all of us. We're doctors. We respect your education and your authority. We're not going to stab you in the back. At least most of us won't. There's only a few of the doctors around whom you must be careful. Your predecessor, Herr

27

Doctor Breit. Herr Doctor Braun, the old fossil. Herr Doctor Miller--he's one of Herr Professor Klein's rats."

"I've met him. Herr Doctor Miller. He seemed friendly until he learned that I was born in Hungary."

"Yes, that sounds like Miller. Both he and Klein are obsessed with nationalities and politics." Doctor Eckhof studied Semmelweis's manner to determine how his new supervisor would react to his familiar tone and to his lack of title for Klein and Miller. He was relieved to see he could continue. Semmelweis might turn out to be a chief resident the young doctors and medical students could trust. "He will continue to report on you for Herr Professor Klein. As he does on all of us."

Doctor Semmelweis wasn't sure whether to trust this doctor he had just met. After the previous day's shocks he wasn't sure he could put his confidence in anyone. But he knew he must discover where the danger was greatest for a Hungarian. "I'm not political. To report on me seems totally unnecessary."

"We all feel that way. This is a medical facility, not a kindergarten. But you have to be aware of the games some doctors play, Herr Doctor."

"Herr Doctor Miller was in Herr Professor Klein's office yesterday before I was admitted. I did have the feeling he felt the need to discuss me before I met with Herr Professor Klein."

"Herr Doctor Miller gave you the introductory tour around the hospital?"

"Yes."

"Herr Doctor Miller is assigned that task by Herr Professor Klein. All of the younger physicians are escorted around the hospital on our first day by Herr Doctor Miller. To uncover any signs of unorthodox politics or philosophy. Klein may have suspected you are not a Conservative and therefore you might not be someone to be trusted. Miller is already convinced you are some kind of heretic, telling everyone in a conspiratorial tone that you're Hungarian. not that most of us care. But to the Conservatives, you were recommended by Herr Doctor Skoda and Baron von Rokitansky. You are regarded by association as an extremely radical person, Herr Doctor Semmelweis."

Doctor Semmelweis grew frightened.

"I jest, Herr Semmelweis. We're all students of Skoda and von Rokitansky, so to speak. We're all doctors or medical students. We're all pledges in the new movement in medicine. Our brotherhood is the modern revolution of the autopsy tables. Von Rokitansky has all of us doing autopsies twenty-four hours a day, seven days a week. I would think your nose would have already informed you of this, Herr Doctor. Only Klein and his toadies don't stink like a sewer. That's how you'll know whom you can trust. If you don't feel like fainting from the smell of a doctor, then be careful what you say to him."

In spite of his distrust, Doctor Semmelweis rewarded Eckhof with a smile.

"Did you say something political to Miller?"

"No."

"But you look so frightened, Herr Doctor. Klein must have given you a severe warning about something. You don't appear to be the timid sort. You must have said something that Miller and Klein interpreted as Liberal. Or is this all because you now believe you cannot be forgiven because you were born in Hungary?"

"I asked about the Second Clinic."

"Unfortunate. You asked about the Second Clinic on your first day at Vienna General Hospital. Very bad, Herr Doctor Semmelweis. Seriously. You should never mention the Second Clinic around the older doctors again, except for Skoda and von Rokitansky. The toady Miller told you that the First Clinic has many more fatalities than the Second Clinic, and so you were curious?"

"He said more than three times as many mothers die in the First Clinic as in the Second. It sounded crazy. I know it can't possibly be true. I wondered why he would say something so unbelievable to a doctor he had just met. And I had heard a woman giving birth outside the window and she was screaming that she did not want to be brought into the hospital, that she didn't want to die, that she knew it was a Death Day."

"Yes, yesterday was a Death Day. And tomorrow. Every other day is a Death Day to the poor mothers of Vienna, because they will have to see a doctor instead of a midwife. We keep a strict discipline in the First Clinic. Go into labor on the wrong day and you get examined by Death itself."

"You're joking again? You're being sarcastic?"

29

"No, it's what these women believe. They would much rather be treated by a midwife than a doctor. The rumor is that it is nearly certain death for a woman giving birth to be assisted by a doctor here. That the Baron wants thousands more dead mothers for his autopsies."

"That's unconscionable. Who would spread such a rumor?"

"We doctors."

"What?"

"We doctors create these stories.. The statistics are sickening. It does appear that the First Clinic is a shortcut to the cemetery."

"I refuse to believe that. And the Second Clinic is better? You can't convince me that what Herr Doctor Miller claims can be true. You can't tell me that a maternity clinic directed by midwives is superior to a clinic where the births are assisted by surgeons."

"Okay, I won't tell you that, Herr Professor Klein. I won't embarrass you with the truth."

"I find what you are implying is very difficult to accept."

"Yes, we should not accept it. We must acknowledge it. Facts are facts, if we are to practice real scientific medicine. We can't ignore what is in front of our eyes."

"Herr Doctor Miller said 240 women died in the First Clinic last year?"

'That number is smaller than the number of women who actually died from childbed fever. We get so many women who come down with the disease that we sometimes we have to take them elsewhere to die."

"Herr Doctor Miller said only 60 women died of childbed fever in the midwives' clinic last year."

"Herr Doctor Miller wants to embarrass the Czech Liberals Professor Baron von Rokitansky and Doctor Skoda by proving their Liberal ideas are a disaster. But Professor Klein has also been conducting the same medical revolution as von Rokitansky and Skoda, so Miller could get caught in his own noose. He may get on the bad side of Klein. But perhaps Miller thinks he will be the next director of the First Clinic, that he will shame old Klein out of his position and take his place."

"So the idea that Herr Doctor Miller is spreading, that the midwives clinic is superior to the doctors' clinic, is just a sneaky gambit?"

"Of course our clinic is superior. We're doctors and medical students. There are only midwives in the Second Clinic."

"So its not true that only one-fourth as many mothers died in the midwives' clinic as in our clinic?"

"No, that's true."

"What?"

"It's true. The Second Clinic had far fewer deaths than our clinic."

"I find that hard to believe."

"As do we all, Herr Doctor Semmelweis. The First Clinic usually has at least three or four times as many deaths per month as the midwives' maternity clinic. Sometimes six times as many, sometimes ten times as many,"

"Do you mean to say there are sometimes ten more deaths a month in the First Clinic?"

"No, I meant to say sometimes ten times *as many* as in the midwives' clinic."

"Then there has to be some scientific reason for the difference. Is there something you are leaving out of the story, Herr Doctor Eckhof? In the First Clinic we must have many more patients. That might be why the death rate is so high. Because of the overcrowding. You did say we get so many mothers here that sometimes they must be taken elsewhere to die?

"And of course the First Clinic must get all the difficult cases. Midwives are not going to be allowed to do births when the baby is arriving head first, am I right? It stands to reason we would have more childbed fever here. That has to be the reason so many more mothers die in the First Clinic. There has to be some logical reason like the type of maternity cases we doctors accept. Or perhaps its because of overcrowding. Or this terrible heat. The Second Clinic probably doesn't have all these patients crowded together. I am correct in my assumptions, am I not?"

"No, Herr Doctor Semmelweis. Do you think you are the first to ask these questions? The midwives in the Second Clinic naturally see approximately the same number of patients as we doctors since on alternate days patients are selected for one or the other clinic. Actually, the Second Clinic would probably have double the number of women giving birth, if we allowed incoming patients their preference. The poor women of Vienna call the days that mothers are sent to the First Clinic 'Death Days'."

"Yes, I've already learned that."

"There's quite a bit of truth in that term."

"The whole notion seems so illogical. So unscientific. I can't believe it. There must be some causative factor that has been overlooked."

"Then it has been overlooked for nearly half a decade. The maternity clinic was separated into a doctors' clinic and a midwives' clinic five years ago, so that midwives could be trained separately from the new doctors. The previous arrangement was distracting and confusing for both doctors and midwives, I am told."

"The separation into two maternity clinics makes sense. But the assertion or the idea that midwives could be five or ten times more successful than medical school graduates...that is worse than absurd."

"Perhaps. We'll see. You're in charge of keeping the numbers now, Semmelweis. It was Herr Doctor Breit's job. But since you're Breit's replacement, you'll be keeping the tally. Let's go to Breit's old office. It will probably be your office now. I'll show you where they keep track of the fatalities for both clinics. But never mention the Second Clinic to your predecessor, Herr Doctor Breit, or to Herr Professor Klein or any of his rats. It's a terrible embarrassment to them, to say the least. Actually, the numbers shame all of us. You couldn't have known it, Doctor Semmelweis, but you couldn't have made a worse mistake than asking about the Second Clinic yesterday. Even being a Hungarian is a secondary offense to uttering aloud the curse words, 'Second Clinic'."

"I don't think any doctor has a need to run away from what he observes. We need to confront this abnormal discrepancy between the clinics, not hide it. If indeed there is such an enormous difference between the death rates."

"Herr Doctor Semmelweis, with all due respect, the topic of the First Clinic is a forbidden one. Herr Professor Klein and the doctors who have been here the longest will despise you if you bring up the subject in front of them."

Doctor Semmelweis was extremely skeptical that a clinic run by doctors could be less effective than one staffed by midwives. Yet he let Doctor Eckhof lead him to Doctor Breit's old office. Did Eckhof have some ulterior motive? Was he some Liberal trying to lure Semmelweis into the war game that seemed to be on-going in the clinic? Nevertheless, Semmelweis was too curious about the death rate numbers to not follow Eckhof, who left him with the piles of statistics he had inherited.

The record-keeping was meticulous, although Doctor Semmelweis still recalled that the doctor who had given him his first-day tour had remarked that Semmelweis's predecessor, Herr Doctor Franz Breit, had omitted statistics for mothers who had been taken elsewhere to die.

Even if this omission were true, the death rates of mothers giving birth in the First Clinic were, to Semmelweis, staggering. Up to the beginning of July the mortality percentage for 1846 was over 10%.

"Is this the way medicine is supposed to be?" the young surgeon mumbled aloud.

Many more patients had been admitted in the first half of 1846 than in previous years. Was overcrowding the reason for so many deaths?

Doctor Semmelweis searched the previous years' records. In 1845 the First Clinic had had approximately 3500 patients with an official mortality rate of nearly 7%. In 1844 3157 patients had been admitted with a death rate of 8.2%. In 1843 3,060 patients and the rate was 9%. In 1842 3287 mothers-to-be had come to the First Clinic and 15.8% had died. There were no numbers for the mothers that Doctor Miller had mentioned, who had contracted childbed fever and who had been moved elsewhere to die.

So the epidemic of childbed fever in the First Clinic was not a recent abnormality. And all the doctors seemed to be aware of this plague, though some would not speak of it.

Sweet Lord, Semmelweis swore to himself, is this medicine?

From that moment until his last breath Herr Doctor Ignaz Semmelweis would be obsessed with the epidemic of childbed fever and its causes.

Chapter Four

The following day was a Death Day and the First Clinic was busy. Doctor Semmelweis first made the rounds of patients, taking notes and preparing the way for Professor Klein. On this day he would finally accompany the director of the First Clinic and introduce each patient's case history to Professor Klein. But what was he allowed say? Was it as forbidden to speak of childbed fever as it was to mention the Second Clinic? The agony of childhood fever was everywhere, and it was almost as unbearable for the young Doctor Semmelweis as it was for the dying mothers.

Now he himself wondered why these women would allow themselves to be brought here. Was the pain of giving birth so terrible that they would allow themselves the risk of this terrible plague? Did they just not realize what terrible danger they were in? Hadn't they been warned by friends who had given birth in the First Clinic? Even the mothers who had escaped unscathed from the bowels of the First Clinic must have described this Eighth Circle of Hell to others in Vienna after they had left the First Clinic. Why would any patient come here? Hadn't they heard the expression 'Death Day'?

Other doctors had affirmed to Semmelweis that most of these women had showed no signs of disease when they had been brought into the First Clinic. That news had sickened Doctor Semmelweis. That could not be! Doctors could not be the cause of the disease, as some mothers-to-be believed. That whole idea was insane.

Herr Doctor Rosenberg had told Semmelweis the story he had already heard several times, "Yes, Herr Doctor Semmelweis. The women who give birth in the street almost never come down with childbed fever."

"That makes no sense," Semmelweis had protested to no one in particular again and again.

Herr Doctor Eckhof had agreed with his friend, Rosenberg, "But it's true, Herr Doctor Semmelweis. Sadly, it's true. Women who give birth in the street and then are admitted to the First Clinic almost never contract childbed fever."

"In England they claim that childbed fever is contagious," Doctor Rosenberg added. "The Englander Oliver Wendell Holmes says that's the reason women giving birth at home don't contract the disease."

"What does that have to do with street births being safer? If that is true, that sick women are contagious, then women giving birth in the street should get childbed fever after they are given a bed here. They would contract childbed fever from the other women in this clinic. And what is it about the street-birthing women that would maintain their four humours in balance? Nothing. What is it about giving birth in the First Clinic that would throw the other women's humours so far out of equilibrium as to damn them quickly with a fatal disease? The Englander's hypothesis has no logic, no basis in scientific observation."

Could something in the First Clinic itself be fatally affecting the humours of women? For this to be true, it would have to condemn them only if they came into the clinic before they gave birth or when they were giving birth. It seemed that Death passed over most of those who came to the First Clinic after giving birth. That shouldn't be happening. That explanation itself didn't conform to scientific medicine.

Doctor Semmelweis did not believe that bad air or some factor of contagion could be the cause of childbed fever. Women who entered the clinic after giving birth almost never contracted the disease. They breathed the same air. They were around the other mothers.

No one familiar with the clinic blamed the clinic itself for the epidemics. Impoverished women in Vienna believed that the First Clinic was a safe place to take to childbed *if they had already given birth.* This could be regarded as a superstitious belief, but it was also good science. The poor mothers of Vienna had *observed* that women who entered the clinic after giving birth survived. They had *concluded* that a Death Day was only a death day if a woman hadn't given birth yet. The reluctant conclusions of embarrassed doctors and of five years' worth of relieved mothers seemingly had established this verity. How then could the new chief resident find any flaw in the conclusions everyone had already drawn? It wasn't the other mothers. It wasn't the clinic itself. The unavoidable fact was--childbed fever must have something to do with the doctors.

Or maybe not. Maybe there was another idea that made more sense. Perhaps it was fate. Perhaps these women were supposed to die. That was one terrible inference some people drew from the years of data. Was the process of birth itself only for certain classes of women? Was the Lord Himself sending a message that only women of privilege should populate the earth?

35

Semmelweis had been trained as a compassionate humourist. He would not allow himself to surrender to the idea that he was the agent by which the Creator ensured that only 'better' women increased the population. And yet he had heard some doctors espouse this idea.

What shameful ideas some doctors propagated. If Semmelweis was now only God's executioner, medicine no longer made sense to him. It wasn't conforming to science. It was not bending to logic.

What made his third day at work bearable to Doctor Semmelweis was the idea that he expected to meet with his good friend, Herr Doctor Jakob Kolletschka later in the evening. So many questions now tortured Semmelweis. Perhaps Jakob could answer them. He would not have to hold his tongue nor censor his scientific curiosity for Kolletschka. He would not have to withhold his feelings in the company of his friend.

"I will see my friend tonight," Semmelweis repeated like a mantra all that third day. The thought made the young man much stronger.

The head of the First Clinic was civil that morning as he and Doctor Semmelweis moved from patient to patient. Doctor Semmelweis felt no adverse reaction each time he'd mention that a mother had childbirth fever. He felt relieved that the disease itself seemed to carry no political connotations. He had even asked Doctors Eckhof and Rosenberg what was the proper term for the disease when addressing Doctor Klein or other Conservatives, which had greatly amused them.

"It's not the disease that bothers them," Eckhof had assured Semmelweis. "It's the embarrassment that a clinic run by midwives has a much better reputation than the First Clinic. You can talk about the disease, but never mention the Second Clinic nor the bad numbers. It's devastating to all of us, but more so to Klein, Braun, and other Conservatives. They like to blame the Liberals, particularly Baron von Rokitansky and Joseph Skoda. But everyone feels stained by the deaths. We are all a part of the revolution in medicine, and are expected to have better outcomes."

"I could never say a bad word about Herr Doctor Skoda or Herr Doctor von Rokitansky."

"Don't. Don't do that. It would gain you nothing. And Klein would see right through you. He believes in scientific medicine, too. He respects the revolution in medicine. He's been a part of it for more than two decades. Be yourself, Semmelweis. That's my advice. Be yourself. Don't try to live with two faces."

Doctor Semmelweis felt no need to compromise his honor that day. He spent his time with Professor Klein that morning limiting his speech to the minimum needed to fulfill his duties as chief resident and assistant to Professor Klein. He spoke very carefully and this could not have gone unnoticed by his superior.

The wall of suspicion between Semmelweis and the Professor was already wider, taller and thicker than any other relationship that Semmelweis was developing in the hospital. Doctor Semmelweis despaired of their being any path through or around the tension. He would have to learn to endure the demeaning role the Professor had picked for him. Klein seemed to delight in demonstrating by tone of voice and gesture how his new chief resident was already skating on thin ice.

In the afternoon Semmelweis supervised an autopsy of a woman who had died of childbed fever, despite the terrible heat in the clinic, and immediately afterward he helped two healthy women give birth. He had found no obvious clue to the epidemic during the autopsy.

In the evening he explained this to his friend, Doctor Kolletschka.

Doctor Kolletschka expressed his own frustration. "There are so many ways for the four humours to be imbalanced. There are so many possibilities. Even though the world recognizes that Baron von Rokitansky, Doctor Skoda, and Doctor von Hebra have been leading a scientific revolution at Vienna General Hospital, it is also aware that we are no closer to finding the solution to the childbed fever epidemic than four thousand autopsies ago. If the revolution in medicine is to prove its worth, we must find the clue to what causes these fevers. And that battle has seemed like fighting a monster with a thousand arms. Perhaps there are a hundred different branches of childbed fever. Maybe the combination of factors that cause mothers to die is too complex for even science to decipher."

"There may be a hundred types of fevers we have lumped into one category?"

"It's possible. Was the woman whom you autopsied bled correctly? Was her doctor's technique satisfactory?"

"Yes, just as we were all taught at the University of Vienna."

"Then she received the proper medical care, Ignaz. Sometimes we doctors can do nothing."

"The number of fatalities doesn't seem excessive to you?"

"Of course it does. It may get worse in the autumn. My understanding is that during the summer the death rate is lower than in colder months. You said last August and June through October two years ago the rates were very low?"

"Yes, but not this summer. The death rate was over 10% in June and over 13% in May this year."

"Perhaps the numbers are unreliable. I think, though, rather than questioning your predecessor's records, it might be more prudent to insure that your own number-keeping is meticulous. Wait a while. Wait, and draw your conclusions from your notes alone. You're going to have to be very patient, my friend, and you and I both know that patience is not one of your virtues. You're going to have to be a sharp observer. Let the solution come to you. You're very earnest. Maybe sometimes you are too driven, but because you care so much about eradicating disease, perhaps the forces that control the world of thought will lead you to a solution. You know, of course, that doctors have battled childbed fever for centuries."

"I saw that the terrible numbers recorded in the First Clinic go back into the last century. I had no idea the epidemic was so bad. I find it incredible that such a disease has raged for so long. It seems that Herr Baron von Rokitansky or Herr Doctor Skoda or some other brilliant man would have found a solution by now."

"Perhaps Herr Doctor Ignaz Semmelweis will save the mothers of the world."

"I am not of that conceit, Jakob. I cannot believe I could uncover some clue that Herr Baron von Rokitansky and Herr Doctor Skoda did not see. Certainly I have not the kind of expertise that my professors have. And I have not the kind of experience that you have, Jakob. You have performed hundreds of autopsies. You must have seen some similarity in all the mothers that died of childbed fever."

"I am sorry to disappoint you, my friend. I have not. No one has. Otherwise we would already have stopped the mothers from dying."

"What good am I, Jakob? It seems the mothers of Vienna would be much better off if all we doctors quit the birthing rooms, and left the task forever to midwives."

"The screams of the dying have disheartened you, my friend. Do you question your choice of profession?"

"Yes. Herr Professor Klein told me that he became director of the First Clinic after his predecessor quit. Herr Professor Klein said his predecessor was so depressed by the number of women who were dying under his care that he no longer wanted to go on. Then he told me something I would never have expected to hear from him. He told me the death rate is much higher than when his predecessor quit, and always has been. Despite the fact that Herr Professor Klein instituted scientific medical practices after he became director. He conducted autopsy after autopsy, exactly as Herr Professor von Rokitansky or you would have done. An Austrian Conservative confessed this to a Hungarian."

"That was a startling admission on the Herr Professor's part."

"I suppose he knew I would discover the fact. I am in charge of the record-keeping. But it haunts me that he has done exactly as any good doctor should, and yet the death rate has climbed. It became much worse only a few months after he had become director and it has stayed high. Should I believe that Herr Professor Klein has not been practicing scientific medicine, as he swears?"

"His quarrel with Herr Professor von Rokitansky and Herr Doctor Skoda is about politics, not about medicine. There are ten thousand opinions about politics in Vienna, but only one view of medicine."

"I do not understand how, after more than two decades, scientific medicine has not discovered what is killing these women. I do not think I will be able to sleep tonight. I feel so agitated. There were times today that I thought the cries of the mothers would drive me insane."

"Good. Let it motivate you. Let the dying spur you to save the living. Vienna General Hospital is at the forefront of a scientific revolution in medicine. If ever there is a location where the solution to this disease is to be found, it will be here in Vienna. Do your autopsies carefully, my friend. Conduct your postmortems exactly as you were taught. Our leaders, Herr Professor von Rokitansky and Herr Doctor Skoda will lead us in this new age of scientific diagnosis. Don't become discouraged. You should be excited to be part of such an advanced movement. We're all going to be famous, you know. Don't get frustrated so easily. Think of the future. It's only your third day."

"I am confounded. After decades of this revolution in medicine, why would the midwives have better results than trained surgeons?"

"I don't know, my friend."

"Jakob, I've copied down the numbers of the mothers who died in the two clinics since 1841. That's when the clinics were separated into a doctors' clinic and a midwives' clinic. In 1841 the date rate was 7.8% for the First Clinic, and 3.5% for the Second Clinic. In 1842 15.8% and 7.6%. In 1843 it was 9% and 6%. In 1844 and 1845 the difference was even more unbelievable. It was 8.2 % in the First Clinic in 1844 and 2.3 % in the Second Clinic. In 1845 it was 6.9% but again only 2% in the Second Clinic."

"I'm sure there's no conspiracy to kill mothers, Ignaz."

"No, of course not. But what could cause such a discrepancy? Both clinics had approximately the same number of admissions, so I don't think overcrowding is the cause. Also, if the fever is spread from mother to mother shouldn't both clinics have about the same number of fatalities?"

"That seems logical."

"Can you think of any reason why there should be three times as many women dying of childbed fever in the First Clinic?"

"I've already said I don't know, Ignaz."

"But you can guess how important these numbers are. If we can discover what this mysterious difference between the clinics is, perhaps we have the key to not only curing childbed fever, but many other diseases as well. What do you know of Herr Professor Franz Klein? Is he really to be angered by anyone who feels we should investigate this difference in death rates between the two clinics?"

"I think you should tread carefully around Professor Klein, Ignaz. But not too cautiously, or he will think you do not have as much favor with Herr Baron von Rokitansky and Herr Doctor Skoda as he fears. Professor Klein may be director of the First Clinic but he knows who recommended you for your position. He must champion his own position and politics but he does not want to run afoul of any of the men of great reputation in Vienna General Hospital. You can use your connections from medical school to protect yourself. However, for the time being I'm afraid, you should limit your curiosity about these numbers you are showing me. Wait and observe."

Doctor Jakob Kolletschka smiled fondly at his friend. He knew Semmelweis was emotional and prone to alternate bouts of great enthusiasm and depression. He worried for Semmelweis because he was very often impatient, and that was a dangerous trait in Habsburg Vienna. He wanted to counsel Semmelweis against talking to others about the difference in death rates between the First Clinic and the Second Clinic, but he knew that Semmelweis was a great comet. Nothing would change his orbit. Nothing would stand in his destined path. He only hoped that some day his friend would not suddenly crash to earth.

It did not surprise Doctor Kolletschka when he heard two months later from his friend that Semmelweis was about to throw caution to the wind and take his numbers to the giant who loomed over Vienna General Hospital, the world-renowned Baron Carl von Rokitansky.

Chapter Five

Baron Carl von Rokitansky, the Colossus of Vienna General Hospital, Czech surgeon, proponent of the new Liberalism sweeping the continent of Europe, politician, humanist, leader of the new revolution in medicine. Untouchable?

"Young Semmelweis the firebrand," the Baron greeted the young doctor who had been chief resident at Vienna General Hospital's First Clinic less than eight weeks. After a pause and a wince from Semmelweis the Baron added, "But Herr Professor Kolletschka has informed me that you are trying very hard to behave, that you have exhibited perfect discipline around the Conservatives. Your friend is very worried about you, Semmelweis. He is afraid you are going to damage your career.

"And well he should be, Semmelweis. Your superior claims that on your first day you were already asking about the Second Clinic. Are you trying to undermine Herr Professor Klein? Are you ambitious, Semmelweis? Are you a Cassius trying to undo the Caesar of the First Clinic?"

"No, Herr Professor, I certainly am not. I am the same as when I was your student, Herr Baron. I am still your loyal student, in fact. It is only that I heard a woman in labor screaming about not wanting to see any doctors. It confounded me that she would rather have midwives assist her delivery. Herr Doctor Miller, who was showing me around the hospital, told me, in fact, that the midwives' clinic has a much better mortality rate than our own clinic."

"He told you that? Semmelweis, you've gotten your first lesson in hospital politics. Herr Doctor Miller is ambitious. He reported you that same day to Herr Professor Klein."

"Yes. I have already assumed as much. Herr Professor Klein expressed his displeasure to me that same day. I have sworn not to concern myself with the Second Clinic."

"But secretly you're gathering statistics on both the First and Second Clinic? Some young colleague is surreptitiously obtaining data for you? You didn't know if you could trust the numbers of your predecessors? The results seemed so outlandish? You need to create your own charts? Information that you can trust absolutely. Have I guessed correctly how you are managing to cope with suppressing your urge to investigate the death rate numbers?"

Doctor Semmelweis felt chastened. "I'm quite sorry, Herr Baron."

"No need to apologize, Semmelweis. Quite the contrary. The University of Vienna taught you proper scientific technique. It showed you how to perform an autopsy but it did not prepare you for the suffering and lingering death you see every day. The maternity ward certainly was not your choice of specialty. You were forced to it if you wanted to stay a physician. You been placed in the most excruciating ward in Vienna General Hospital. Now you feel, because you are a surgeon, it is your duty to find the cause of the mothers' fevers.

"You've adjusted to your station, but you don't want to feel useless. You want to do the best you can, even if your present situation is abhorrent to you. You need to make sense of your new life. You must fight your feelings of terrible despair, Herr Doctor Semmelweis. To do that you must help these mothers. That is the source of your ambition, if anyone should label your motives with such a slur. I do not need any informants, like Professor Klein. I know how the various ways doctors and medical students meet their challenges. You fit in the category of needing to be conscientious. You are not going to be satisfied with just your position. I know your soul, Herr Doctor Semmelweis."

Semmelweis nodded.

"I was a young surgeon once. I know the anguish you young doctors must feel. Do you think that I, too, am not frustrated that the revolution in scientific medicine has not found the sources of this terrible disease? To me, Semmelweis, your concern indicates that these dying mothers are real people to you, not leather dress mannequins to be dissected on the autopsy table. They're human to you, Herr Doctor, or you would not care. And I, too, Herr Doctor, am above all things a humanist.

"I am quite aware of what the poor women of Vienna say about me. They claim everywhere that I want more dead mothers for the autopsy tables. But those terrified women have reversed cause and effect. I want more autopsies so there will be fewer dead mothers. That is the truth about our medical revolution here in Vienna, Herr Doctor Semmelweis. I want more autopsies so there will be fewer dead mothers.

"I began like you, Herr Doctor. I am also an idealist. The suffering of these women was real to me, and it did not matter what was their station in life. And, in truth, the knowledge that we gain from our medical revolution will benefit the Empress as much as the prostitute.

"That is why we have greatly increased the numbers of autopsies under my direction, Semmelweis. I am not a butcher. I am not a murderer. I am not some sick experimenter. Like you I want to find the cause of this terrible epidemic that has existed for centuries. I do not believe these women are doomed since birth. I do not believe that Our Lord is punishing these mothers for their sins. I am a humanist, Herr Doctor. I am a scientist. I believe in reason.

"Unfortunately, modern science is complicated. We know that all disease is caused by an imbalance in one or more of the four humours. When I was your age, I was convinced that we could cure childbed fever by examining the liver, where the humour of blood is formed; the spleen, where the humour of yellow bile is invented; the gall bladder, where the black bile originates; and the brain and lungs, where phlegm is formed. I did not think it would take much time to find the cause of diseases. We just needed to do many more autopsies and relate the disease to the organ which had an imbalance of a particular humour.

"We were quite clever in our science. The first question, of course, as I have lectured, is determining what is a healthy organ. If we want to discover the imbalance of a particular humour--whether it is blood, phlegm, yellow bile or black bile--we must first be sure what the parameters of a fully functioning organ can be. How much blood, phlegm, yellow bile, or black bile is healthy? At what point of excess or deficit does the organ begin to malfunction? Does a temporary imbalance have a permanent effect? If not, how long before an imbalanced organ causes systemic damage that cannot be corrected? Should the amounts of a particular humor vary according to age, height, weight, nationality, geographical area, climate, altitude, season?

"I have no need to continue. You were my student. You were the student of Herr Doctor Skoda. I believe you understand that we have greatly increased the number of autopsies because we have found that the task is much more complicated than we had first realized. Perhaps we were all guilty at first of believing that we would open up new mothers who had just died of childbed fever and find that each one of them had an excess of bile. Then we would interview the families to discover if all the victims had the same diet, or came from the same neighborhood, had the same religious practices, and so on. We were naive, Semmelweis. The years have not been kind in yielding the secrets to these diseases. But we can't just give up. We must adhere to our science and its methods. It's all we have.

"I can see your impatience, Semmelweis. I have not told you anything new. You have been searching already for the particular imbalance of humours that causes childbed fever. You have diligently been conducting autopsies. The procedures have only intensified your bewilderment. It is the same for all of us, Herr Doctor.

"But you also believe the answer lies in finding some difference between the profiles of the patients or the practitioners of the First Clinic and Second Clinic. This now interests you more than your autopsies. You wonder if there is something about the air, or the location, or some other factor that has been previously overlooked. It makes no sense to you that midwives should be better doctors than doctors themselves. You want to know what the midwives are doing differently, or what is different about their share of mothers that are admitted to the two clinics. You are, of course, not the first surgeon to ask this question"

"Herr Professor, does it not seem that the secret to childbed fevers could be revealed by finding the critical difference between the doctors' clinic and the midwives' clinic?"

"Your friend, Herr Professor Kolletschka, has explained to me your obsession with the Second Clinic. I, too, once believed that the magic key to saving mothers was hidden somewhere in the midwives' clinic. We have searched and searched, Herr Doctor Semmelweis, and of course we have found nothing that midwives are doing better than doctors. What folly it was to expect that midwives could give better care to mothers-to-be than the most excellent surgeons.

"But you will not be satisfied until you investigate the Second Clinic yourself. Just as you would not have been convinced about the difference in death rates until you kept your own statistics.

"I believe I am about to surprise you, Herr Doctor Semmelweis, I am going to reverse the decision of your superior. I will tell Herr Professor Klein that you will be permitted to investigate the Second Clinic in any way that you see fit, as long as you first dedicate yourself to the duties of chief resident. You will prepare rounds for the director of the First Clinic, conduct autopsies, continue your teaching duties. You are not to diminish in any way your routine responsibilities. You will then be permitted to observe any procedure or interview any personnel in the Second Clinic, as long as they are not a visitor who is your superior. Is this agreeable to you?"

45

"Yes. Of course. Thank you, Herr Baron."

"I sincerely wish you good fortune in your investigation. Perhaps a fresh pair of eyes and a less weary brain will achieve a breakthrough. I have assured Herr Professor Klein that you are not trying to humiliate him and that you will not embarrass him in any way in any future. You will be Herr Professor's Klein loyal assistant without fault. I have told him that he will share equally in any credit for your discoveries. I will have your word as a gentleman on these promises before you leave my office today. Also, I have one more instruction for you, Herr Doctor Semmelweis. It is necessary that you listen carefully to what I have to say.

"No one can predict the changes that will take place in the next few years in Europe. The status of the Habsburg Empire is volatile, as you as a Hungarian, are well cognizant. I myself believe that we will be witness to movements that will transform the entire civilized world for centuries to come. Historians and common citizens alike will cite the mid-nineteenth century as the beginning of a new era for mankind. We live in propitious times, and even surgeons must hold tight to their cap in the midst of the great winds that are brewing.

"You are Hungarian, Herr Doctor. Do not try to pretend to yourself that that does not matter here in the most enlightened city on the continent. Never forget you are Hungarian and not Austrian. No one else will. Suspicion will always be directed toward you, and no one can protect against the forces of prejudice. People in Vienna are fearful. Not just Hungarians, but Czechs, Poles, Italians, Romanians, Serbs, Croats, Slovaks, and even Austrian Germans speak fervently of independence and even of the superiority of their race over the Austrians. Vienna is afraid. Vienna is the capital of the Habsburg Empire and that ruling force is poised to break into a dozen pieces. And each of those pieces must fracture again into even smaller divisions, since all these nationalist movements cannot agree on what type of citizenry and government to which they should aspire.

"People in Vienna are afraid of chaos. They see a terrible tempest on the horizon. They see all that all they hold dear is in jeopardy. Anyone who is not Austrian seems to wish the end of the Austrian Empire, and Austrians are sure they all speak in whispers of this when they are not in earshot of a citizen loyal to the Habsburg future. You will be a threat to Austrian Conservatives no matter how unpolitical you try to appear. Never forget that."

"Yes. Herr Professor."

"You have already stepped heavily on some toes, Herr Doctor Semmelweis.
I know how the mind of doctors can be blind to everything but the finding the
causes of a disease. But courtesy and respect for other doctors are important.
Never make any one of your superiors or colleagues feel like you are
threatening their reputation again. That will not only affect you, but also
your teachers. Since I and Herr Doctor Skoda recommended you, if you ever
make someone at Vienna General Hospital feel that you are disdainful of
their medical knowledge, expertise, or recommendations, they will be
petitioning us to redress such grievances."

"Yes, Herr Professor."

"Now swear to me that you will keep sacred everything I have recommended
today."

"Yes, Herr Baron."

"I wish your investigation the greatest of success."

"Thank you, Herr Baron."

Chapter Six

In the weeks that followed his meeting with his former medical school professor Doctor Semmelweis worked diligently so as not to disappoint his inspiration and benefactor, Baron von Rokitansky. He attended to his duties as chief resident, was enthusiastic in his teaching responsibilities and more than met his quota of autopsies.

It should not have disappointed him that he could not pinpoint an excess or deficit of one particular humour in the mothers who had succumbed to childbed fever. Many surgeons before Doctor Semmelweis had not found any glaring similarities among the mothers who had given birth and then had died sometimes only days later. The leader of the new revolution in scientific medicine himself, Baron von Rokitansky had already explained that his own efforts had thus far been in vain. Why should the young Semmelweis have expected to reverse the failures of all those who had come before him? What deluded vanity had led Semmelweis to believe that he could do better than those who had previously inspired him? Yet he felt almost a panic, an urgency to rid himself of his new self-image as a failure. Moreover, he could not allow Vienna to doubt its doctors. He and his clinic must banish the idea of Death Days and of doctors as God's executioners, and quickly.

Death Days! Doctor Semmelweis could not allow that medicine which he knew was the salvation of his patients to be classified as their doom, no more than a priest could allow his parish to believe that Jesus had been the Devil. This term 'Death Days' recalled the superstitious Vienna of the past, which had believed that many diseases were caused by the vampire bat. In fact this notion had not yet been fully banished in some strata of society. Strange ideas from the by-gone days were still afloat. Only scientific medicine could exile these misconceptions and keep them from returning. Death Days indeed! Civilization depended on doctors proving that the future should belong to science.

New peculiar notions were also being born inside the fractures of European societies. In the Vienna of 1846 paranoia was reaching a fever pitch as the minorities within the Austrian Empire realized they could not settle for the compromises of the past. No one was happy with the economic and political situation. The dissatisfaction led to the kind of emotional charges that lacked fairness and reflection. The time was one in which people on all sides of an issue seemed to want to vent their frustration much more than find a solution to it. The First Clinic was the subject of many vicious rumors on the streets of Vienna. Many of the younger doctors under Semmelweis's direction felt afraid of being accused of anti-humanist feelings, of not caring whether poorer mothers lived or died. A paranoia was increasing within and without the First Clinic.

Irrational demands seemed to be flourishing while rational debate was in decline. Doctor Semmelweis feared at times that logic might not command in the general population the position it deserved unless he found a way to assert its rightful dominance. He saw everywhere a self-indulgence that paid no heed to the long-term effect of its pettiness, and it scared him. What if this extreme carelessness took hold? Modern medicine might fail miserably and give way to the ignorance of the past. Scientific medicine might be forever doomed if the doctors at Vienna General Hospital could not give some rationale for the thousands of postmortems, if they could not find some startling discovery to justify their experiments.

And yet, most other doctors, Semmelweis sometimes thought, seemed strangely unconcerned, almost arrogant, as if their behavior was so far above the questions of ordinary Viennese that they didn't need to give it a thought. In contrast Semmelweis believed that their moment to establish the new revolution with unarguable permanence was quickly fading. He felt a great burden on his shoulders. Could Vienna General Hospital become the great dam that held back the flood of ignorance? Only if Semmelweis found a solution to childbed fever. Only if mothers stopped dying in the doctors' clinic. Only if the term 'Death Day' became a relic of a past age.

Semmelweis needed to find the solution that had eluded his teachers. If only there were something simple that had been overlooked. If only every mother that had died after childbirth displayed too much blood in her liver, too little black bile in her gall bladder, or too much phlegm in her lungs. But no matter how many autopsies, no one single factor proclaimed itself as the parent of childbed fever.

In July 1846 Doctor Semmelweis recorded the deaths of 33 mothers who had earlier given birth in the First Clinic. The mortality rate was 13.1% In August, in Doctor Semmelweis's second month as chief resident, the already horrifying rate climbed even further, to 18.1%. In September and October the rate of deaths was between 14-15% in both months.

Nothing explained the fever. Women whose birth Semmelweis had personally assisted and whom he had isolated to observe if some clinic contagion was a factor still often died. These same women had also not been subject to the environmental factors of the First Clinic and yet they had succumbed.

One prominent doctor in particular had insisted that there were dozens of causes to childbed fever, that the contagion had endured for so many years precisely because there was no one cause. Was this idea valid? If so, they might never be able to prevent mothers from dying of these fevers.

Doctor Semmelweis spent as much of his free time as possible observing the Second Clinic, interviewing the relatives of victims, watching the midwives at work, searching every corner of the birthing rooms and the wards, watching how the beds were prepared, how the sheets were laundered, even how the midwives addressed their patients. Not even the most minute detail of the midwives' daily routine escaped his examination.

"I can find no critical differences at all between the clinics," he complained to his best friend, Doctor Kolletschka. Yet the Second Clinic still consistently had a death rate for mothers who had recently given birth that was one-third or one-fourth or even less that that of the First Clinic.

"It is not unexpected that the practices of the midwives are the same as those of the doctors," Doctor Kolletschka, a professor of forensic medicine at the hospital, sympathized. "After all, they were trained by the doctors here. It's not surprising that you find no statistical differences between the eating habits, the religious customs, the daily routines, or any factor between the patients in both clinics. They are, after all, selected only because of their day of arrival at the clinic. You might as well be trying to distinguish between the personal habits of Wednesday and Thursday.

"I'm afraid, my dear friend, you have set an impossible task for yourself." Professor Kolletschka, who was in essence a detective for the causes of disease, who had seen years of discouragement and failure himself, could merely repeat the worn wisdom that was now only an opiate for the defeated army of doctors. "You are attempting to find the answer to one of the greatest medical mysteries of all time. But, of course, we all must keep trying to find a cure. We must stay diligent.

"You look tired. You must find some time away from the clinic, Ignaz. And you must get more sleep."

"I cannot. I cannot bear the prospect of defeat. The deaths haunt my every waking moment and my fitful nights."

In November 1846 the death rate in the First Clinic was 10.8%.

"We could do ten thousand autopsies a day," the frustrated Semmelweis protested to many of the other doctors. "It does no good." Few of them disagreed with Semmelweis's conclusion. Why even bother with so many autopsies? He was aware that he was echoing the recent sentiment of Professor Klein, but perhaps the Professor was correct in becoming disillusioned with the revolution he claimed to have inspired. The autopsies were proving nothing. They were uncovering nothing.

Fortunately, the spiritually exhausted doctors and students of The First Clinic were soon granted a long sabbatical from the study of corpses. By coincidence the assistant of obstetrics who had temporarily replaced Semmelweis in supervising students as they conducted autopsies, and whose looming presence forced students to perform many more postmortems, seldom chose to visit the morgue in December. This was a happy vacation for the medical students, even though they were often eager to learn about anatomy. Most new doctors and medical students followed the example of the autopsy instructor and now only performed the postmortems that were legally required.

Happily for Semmelweis and many other surgeons who had thus far found the postmortems to be an ineffective diagnostic tool, the official was also absent for the beginning months of 1847. For the next four months, until Doctor Semmelweis retook the position as the instructor of autopsies, very few autopsies were done.

Doctor Semmelweis told no one he was becoming disillusioned with the results the autopsies had provided. His lack of diligence in this area must have been reported to the director of the First Clinic. Professor Klein had called Semmelweis into his office one day. "I am sure you know blood has the most influence of the four humours. Have you seen an excess in the women you have autopsied?"

"No, Herr Professor." Doctor Semmelweis only had to think back to the autopsies he had performed in the previous autumn and summer in order to answer the director's question honestly.

"You are bleeding the mothers who are feverish? Those whose genitals are infected?"

"Yes, Herr Professor. We have increased the number of leeches that are

51

being applied to the sick women, exactly as you have suggested."

"This does not improve their condition?"

"No, Herr Professor."

"So the imbalance may be in the spleen or the gall bladder. These women may have an excess of yellow bile or black bile?"

"The autopsies have not shown any such imbalance in these humours."

"So you're saying then, Semmelweis, that it must be an excess of phlegm that is killing these mothers?"

"No, Herr Professor."

"You are aware, Semmelweis," Professor Klein continued in a sarcastic tone, "that there are only four humours? Or have you discovered a fifth?"

"No, Herr Professor."

"Are the women too calm and unemotional? This is the characteristic of an excess of phlegm."

"Most of the mothers scream in pain all day and night, Herr Professor."

"You have tried emetics?"

"Yes, Herr Professor."

"You have increased the genital examinations of the mothers after they have given birth?"

"Yes, Herr Professor. We have greatly increased the number of genital examinations these last two months."

Semmelweis recognized that Klein was in one of his bad moods. "Liberals and foreigners," the Professor pretended to mumble to himself, "are both useless. And my chief resident is both." He looked up at his chief resident. "You're dismissed, Semmelweis."

Doctor Semmelweis realized that this meeting with Klein was just more of the usual harassment that seemed to fulfill Klein's needs for a month or so.

The hastily arranged meetings never accomplished anything except to press home the point that Klein knew it was the fault of his chief resident that so many mothers were dying. However, this day's particular pettiness would save many lives in the future. Doctor Semmelweis would remember Klein's unnecessary questions and use them later as a way to stave off the director's interference in a vital experiment.

In December Professor Klein needed no scapegoat. Just as everyone was convinced the newest increase in childbed fever deaths would never subside, the tragic situation suddenly took a surprising turn.

Doctor Semmelweis announced that half as many mothers had succumbed to childbed fever in December 1846 as in November. The mortality rate was 5.4%, an incredible improvement. The death rate had not fallen below 10% in nearly a year and a half.

In the corridors of Vienna General Hospital there were whispers that Herr Doctor Semmelweis had suddenly begun fudging the statistics.

In early February the chief resident announced an even lower rate of 3.2% for the first month of the new year. The ugly rumors about the chief resident grew.

"The rates vary tremendously from month-to-month," Semmelweis's friends and apologists tried to point out. "They always have."

On the first of March Doctor Semmelweis announced a death rate of 1.6% for February, half of the rate for January. There was a good deal of skepticism about the numbers. Within the First Clinic, though, many doctors knew there had been few fatalities.

That same day Doctor Semmelweis found signs posted in his office.

"Go back to Pest, Hungarian liar." Pest was near Semmelweis's hometown in Hungary.

"Leave science to true gentlemen, Magyar barbarian."

Was he losing the favor of some doctors? Why? They of all people should know that Semmelweis was only reporting the strange reversal in the death rate, not inventing it. In February 1847 only six women of the 312 patients admitted to the First Clinic had died of childbed fever.

The doctors in the First Clinic knew he wasn't forging the statistics. Why would someone believe he could invent the death rate statistic and not be discovered? Who would put such a note on his door?

A miracle had happened. We surgeons should all be proud, he thought. For the first time since he had come to the First Clinic in July, 1846, Semmelweis slept well. He no longer felt tortured by the deaths of so many mothers. Herr Doctor Semmelweis thought everyone should be happy, even if he wasn't sure what had caused the relief.

His superior for once was not one of the doctors lined up against Semmelweis. He did not think Semmelweis had reported false statistics. Professor Klein attributed the decline in fatal fevers to his own genius. "It's the increased bloodletting and postpartum vaginal examinations," Professor Klein explained to Semmelweis. "My recommendations have abated this two-centuries old scourge. I will perhaps write articles on this new cure." Professor Klein was still quite abrupt with his chief resident, but at least he didn't believe Semmelweis had invented the mortality numbers for the previous three months. Perhaps Professor Klein was clandestinely even calculating his own tally to compare with those of his chief resident.

He wants to distance me and take full credit for this cure, Semmelweis thought. He is only pretending to be angry. He knows this improvement came about because I did my tasks diligently. But the suggestions that had created the decline in deaths had come from Professor Klein, Semmelweis conceded to himself. He deserves the credit. Semmelweis hoped this new honor for the Professor might presage a lessening of the tension in the air for him. He believed the Professor had been secretly undermining his position with his students. Perhaps Klein would now feel more secure in his reputation and no longer have a need for such injustices.

Doctor Semmelweis also thought it was a good time to request his first vacation and was pleasantly surprised when Professor Klein granted his request.

"So you think Professor Klein may have found a partial cure for the fevers of mothers in childbed, Ignaz." Semmelweis had come to say goodbye to his friend before he left Vienna.

"Possibly. In February only six women died of childbed fever. Since the beginning of December the number of deaths has gone down, down, down." Semmelweis was happy for the director, for himself, and, above all, for the mothers of Vienna.

"We have had three months of results far better than what we could have wished for. Ever since Professor Klein instructed us to apply more leeches, to effect more purges, to induce more vomiting."

"You are practicing these cures on the healthy mothers?"

"No, of course not, Jakob. Only when the mothers get sick, we apply the leeches. We perform the the other standard treatments only on the women with fevers. As always."

"And this affects the healthy women in what way?"

"Not at all."

"How many of the women with fevers passed away in February?"

"Only six. I told you."

"So the leeches did not actually help them?"

"But the death rate for the First Clinic in February was lower than in almost two years."

"How could that possibly have been caused by the treatments you gave to dying women, if it saved none of them?"

"I don't know, Jakob. I have no idea. Nothing makes sense to me. Nothing has been logical since I became chief resident. I do not want to question this wonderful success."

"You're bending to superstition? You don't believe that applying Professor Klein's suggested treatments to women who die anyway could possibly have kept the death rate low?"

"Perhaps it makes no sense, but it worked. I am happy, Jakob. I am pleased that so few mothers have died this winter. I am tired of losing so many patients. The treatment works. Why should I question it? If women are not dying as they did before, why should I not continue the improvements?"

"They're not improvements. You know that, Ignaz. You're too much of a scientist to accept a coincidence as the long-sought cure."

"I don't know that I am much of anything, Jakob. For the first time I am seeing relatively good results in the First Clinic. The news has gotten better and better for three months. I know that leeches for dying women shouldn't increase the number of healthy women in the vicinity that do not contract fevers. But it does. It makes no sense. But the proof is in the results."

"You are fearful of losing your position, Ignaz? You are trying to pacify Professor Klein?"

"I am tired of my patients dying! I am not sure of anything anymore. I know nothing. How can I possibly question the wisdom of Professor Klein or anyone else? I was foolish to believe I could help anyone."

"You were born in 1818, Ignaz. Professor Klein was born in 1788. Baron von Rokitansky was born in 1804. Doctor Skoda, in 1805. You do not believe you could possibly observe something that men so senior would not already have seen. You are too young a doctor for the terrible task of keeping these mothers from dying. The great doctors must find the answers and tell them to you."

"I have not given up. I need to get away for a while."

"A good idea. This grasping at straws is not like you, Ignaz.

"I know how difficult it is for you to have not found a cure yet, but don't be so impatient. You have not been a doctor for all of the thousand years of frustration you feel inside. You must steel yourself against the sounds of suffering before you can silence disease with its cure. Otherwise your eagerness to find a solution will lead you to a lie. And you will do the mothers of Vienna no service if you unthinkingly embrace superstition or coincidence for comfort. Don't give up on scientific medicine."

"Yes, my mind is clouded, Jakob."

Doctor Semmelweis and Professor Koolletschka said a sad goodbye, and Semmelweis went to Venice for a few weeks to enjoy the privilege of being a gentleman surgeon of the Austrian Empire.

Chapter Seven

On March 2, 1847, Doctor Ignaz Semmelweis left Vienna for Venice. He would spend the next weeks savoring the art treasures of that great city.

Those first two weeks in Venice were a happy time. The childbed fever plague had weighed heavily on Semmelweis for eight months, ever since he had heard the screams of the woman trying to give birth on the street near the First Clinic: "Please, please don't take me to the doctors. I don't want to die. Who will take care of my children? I know today is a Death Day."

"Please don't take me to the doctors," the mother-to-be had cried. "I don't want to die."

But the orderlies *had* taken the woman to the doctors. And she *had* died. She haunted Semmelweis.

Were they doctors or were they executioners? What good was it to be a surgeon, a chief resident in fact, at the most advanced hospital in Europe? What good was it to be a medical school graduate well-versed in the principles of modern scientific medicine? He might as well have diagnosed the feverish new mothers as victims of vampire bat bites. They had died no matter what reason he or some other doctor had scribbled on the autopsy report. Cause of death: "Death".

The scourge against mothers had continued unabated for two centuries. Could the nightmare finally be almost over? Could the director of the First Clinic finally have found the solution? More leeches, daily emetics, enemas, more vaginal examinations. Could this be the beginning of a new age for obstetrics?

Could Professor Klein have finally diminished childbed fever? Could mothers-to-be finally not be afraid that giving birth would be their last act in the midst of God's Creation? Could a pregnancy finally be an occasion for great joy instead of constant fear?

Semmelweis fervently hoped that Professor Klein had finally hit upon the combination of measures that would finally make childbirth safe for women. Perhaps Semmelweis would be rid of the recurring nightmare of the impoverished Mother Mary, who had just given birth to the Baby Jesus, piercing the hospital air with the involuntary sounds of the terrible pain of childbed infection.

These were mothers, not deadly criminals. What kind of Creator would foist such a plague on those least deserving of punishment? What kind of Divine Being cursed a certain class of mothers?

More leeches? Forcing sick mothers to vomit? Forcing those who had childbed fever to evacuate everything in their bowels? This were the steps that had been expected of Doctor Semmelweis? This is what he had needed to do to stop the dying? Semmelweis had made the terrible last days and hours of dying mothers even more agonizing. These palliatives for the dying never saved their lives. But for some unknown reason all these methods had helped to solve the problem. Torturing the dying women had insured that very few healthy mothers had contracted childbed fever.

In this way Doctor Semmelweis hoped they were finally putting an end to childbed fever. But he was also afraid. Professor Kolletschka was right, of course. Professor Klein's solutions made no sense to him. On the other hand, there had been miraculous results. No one could argue otherwise. But all the contradictions that Doctor Semmelweis had battled for eight months were not only not yet explained. The absurdities were intensified. Why was there such a huge gap between the numbers of mothers who died in the First Clinic and the Second Clinic? Why did mothers that delivered in their own home seldom contract the infections that killed mothers in Vienna General Hospital's First Clinic? Why did women who delivered in the street and then were brought to the First Clinic seldom get the fever or the infected genital area or the abdomen painful to the touch?

Previously nothing had made sense, Now, with three months of increasingly good news, with the number of mothers who were succumbing to childbed fever going down, down, down...nothing made sense. Professor Klein might as well have been a sorcerer, waving his magic wand for three months and gradually turning every case of childbed fever to vapor. This was as satisfactory an answer as any to the miracle of the winter of 1846-47.

Doctor Semmelweis had longed for a modern scientific explanation for the cause or causes of childbed fever. He still didn't have one. Perhaps he should be satisfied with the fact that far fewer mothers were now getting sick.

Also, he was tired of thinking about disease. He was in Venice. Was there a more wonderful city in all of Europe? And the art! For more than two weeks he tried to forget about medicine, about his responsibilities, about the First

Clinic. It would be unknown to Semmelweis until his return to Austria, but in his absence an event would occur in Vienna that would eventually change the lives of every mother and every woman in Europe. It would benefit womankind until the end of Creation.

A terrible death would lead to salvation for mothers and women everywhere.

Chapter Eight

In the spring of 1847 the fragmenting of the Habsburg Empire was worsening. It was more than just Liberals against Conservatives. Conservatives railed against the newspapers, which they claimed had a Liberal bias and would weaken the Empire. They were anxious at the influx of foreign ideas, remembering what had occurred after revolutions elsewhere. They feared the universities, their students, and a younger generation that had not enough life experience to understand the necessity of the current restrictions. They disdained what others saw as "advances" and not only prepared to hold the line against changes in the Empire, but to reverse some of the relaxations that had already occurred.

Conservatives therefore began to reject two generations of Age of Enlightenment propositions. They seemed to Liberals to be going backward to the pitfalls of a less just time, but Conservatives believed they saw chaos developing and needed to be proactive, particularly because the weak Emperor did not assure them of maintaining their position in the Empire. Organized religion felt threatened by what they regarded as radical ideas. People who had positions of power and prestige had been warned all their lives against what had happened during the French revolution. Now they were afraid the same type of unbridled mob rule could happen within the Austrian Empire. The Empire itself might be challenged and banished if authority did not react to the slightest challenge with overwhelming intimidation.

Habsburg loyalists felt that the Empire was losing its grip. Its defenses must be strengthened. It needed to conscript more and more soldiers, which meant it needed to collect more and more taxes. This increased tensions, since many people were out of work, and a great many even had difficulty finding enough to eat. While many would not risk the possibility of losing their own hard-earned station in life, others lacked the barest necessities for existence and felt invisible. The people crying 'poverty' seemed to be the wealthiest of the Empire, which further convinced the peasant class and lower class they had nothing to lose by letting university students and professors, including those from the University of Vienna, whom the peasants had distrusted because of their elevated station, represent them. It became these upper middle class youth who first confronted the Conservative front. They did not question the authority of the Emperor. They only asked for certain rights and an easing of hardships for the lower class. They spoke of the kind of compassion and freedom that Enlightenment was supposed to have birthed.

But who were the enemies of Liberalism? It was hard to define the opposition. There were a multitude of viewpoints lumped into the classification of Conservatism. There were seemingly irreconcilable differences between the Conservatives within each nationality of the Austrian Empire. There were many issues that were central to these small pockets of Conservatives and about which they would not compromise. These demands were quietly hated by other Conservatives. There seemed to be as many Conservative factions as there were conservatives.

Liberalism seemed to have a unifying platform. Liberalism appealed to the lower classes and much of the educated middle class. Many Liberals wanted education for the lower classes and peasants, more language instruction (the Empire included more than a dozen languages other than Austrian), and concessions to the nationalities that Vienna controlled. French, Poles, Hungarians, Czechs, Italians, Germans, Croatians, Serbs, Slovaks, Romanians and many others wanted reforms and more control over their traditional territories.

To our age the aims of European Liberalism seem reasonable. The demands by European Liberals in 1847 were far less radical than those outlined in the defining document of the American Revolution. There were no demands for freedom of religion or freedom to write whatever they wished. These kind of rights, which the barbarian continent of America had enjoyed without question for more than half a century, Europeans dared not consider. But peasants, students, and many of the working class began to organize against Austrian hegemony and against conscripted labor and slavery, and to actually speak in whispers of allowing "wages".

Wages! Wages for peasants! And from whose pocket would that money come?

However, there were many other issues that were central to small pockets of reformers and about which they would not compromise. These demands were quietly hated by other Liberals. Under closer examination there seemed to be as many Liberal viewpoints as there were Liberals.

Since Vienna was the capital of the far-reaching and powerful Habsburg Empire, it was a focal point for the divisions that defined mid-nineteenth-century Europe. Doctor Semmelweis, who considered himself above seamy politics, returned to Vienna in late March of 1847 to find that even he was being drawn into the growing storm.

On the morning of March 20th he found a large scrap of paper nailed to the door of his office. His friend's name, Professor Jakob Kolletschka, had been written in large letters and then crossed out. Underneath was written by the same hand, "One less Liberal foreigner. Good riddance."

As Semmelweis was reading this note, Doctor Eckhof was walking in the hallway, spied the chief resident, and greeted him gravely, "Welcome back, Herr Doctor."

Semmelweis, who often spoke in a brusque and businesslike manner, and who was often accused of deliberately ignoring conventional pleasantries, turned, surprised by the tone in Doctor Eckhof's voice. "Did you have something to do with this?" Semmelweis accused, pointing at the note.

"No, Herr Doctor. Of course not."

"What is the meaning of this? Is Herr Professor Kolletschka no longer working in the hospital? Has he gone on a long vacation?"

Eckhof was taken aback. "You haven't heard, Herr Doctor?"

"Haven't heard what? I have been on vacation in Venice, of course."

"Herr Doctor Kolletschka died a week ago."

Because the note on the door had made him suddenly suspicious Semmelweis almost accused Eckhof a second time. The expression of sadness and concern on Eckhof's face convinced Semmelweis that his student was not cruelly joking.

"A week ago? How?"

"He was supervising autopsies, and one of the students nicked Herr Professor Kolletschka's finger with the scalpel he was using on the cadaver."

"And?"

"He became sick, increasingly feverish, and then passed away."

"From a cut on his finger?"

"Yes, Herr Doctor."

"That's preposterous."

"Yes, Herr Doctor. Everyone thinks so. It is a terrible tragedy."

Semmelweis was trying to read the thoughts of Doctor Eckhof. "You're not telling me something. You're hiding something from me."

Eckhof nodded slightly. "I've made an exact copy of the autopsy report. Should I fetch it now?"

"If you please, Eckhof. I'll be in my office."

Semmelweis left the hallway and walked to his desk, and slumped into his chair. His best friend had died from a scalpel cut? Could that be true? But what had not been insanity since he had arrived at Vienna General Hospital? The woman pleading not to be cared for by doctors on his first day as chief resident? The midwives far exceeding trained surgeons in their care of mothers? The inconclusive results of so many hundreds of autopsies? Why should today be any different? For a brief moment the most famous speech of Hamlet, a favorite of medical students, flashed through his mind.

Semmelweis had had only one confidant, only one person whose confidence and serenity had steadied him in all these months in hell. Was it really true that Professor Jakob Kolletschka was dead? Could that be possible?

Dead from a cut on the finger? We are all damned, Semmelweis realized, but we are not allowed to understand we are in hell until it is our proper time. Perhaps it is well and proper, the death of Jakob, Semmelweis thought. Perhaps his friend had been released. Perhaps Jakob was in a much better place.

Instinctively, Doctor Semmelweis reached for the only remaining comfort in his life. Doctor Franz Breit, obstetrician, the physician whom Semmelweis had replaced as chief resident the preceding July, had been keeping the numbers for Semmelweis. Semmelweis saw with satisfaction that the death rate was still very low for the First Clinic. Semmelweis was relieved. Here was something that made sense. The level of care in the First Clinic was greatly improved. Here was something to live for--helping the mothers of Vienna.

Eckhof returned with the autopsy report and handed it to Semmelweis, who motioned for Eckhof to have a seat.

Semmelweis began reading the autopsy description carefully: "Inflammation of the lymphatic vessels and veins of the upper extremity. Inflammation of the lung membranes and chest cavity. Inflammation of the sac around the heart. Inflammation of the membranes of the abdomen and pelvic cavity and of the membranes around the brain. Metastasis in one eye."

He finished his reading, looked up, and glared at Eckhof. "Inflammation of the membranes of the abdomen and pelvic cavity. Metastasis in one eye. Inflammation of the lymph vessels, the veins of the upper extremity... Should I go on? This is your idea of a joke?"

"No, Herr Doctor."

"What do you mean by this outrage?"

"Nothing, Herr Doctor."

"Herr Professor Kolletschka was supervising an autopsy of a mother who had died of childbed fever?"

"Yes, Herr Doctor."

"This are the exact autopsy results of a woman dead of childbed fever."

"Yes, Herr Doctor."

"Herr Professor Kolletschka is named as the deceased. You have put my friend's name on the report of a woman dead of childbed fever."

"No, Herr Doctor. I swear to you, that *is* the autopsy report for Herr Professor Kolletschka. We are all shocked. We do not know what it means. Perhaps the English have been right all along. Perhaps we have been dealing with a contagious disease these last two centuries. Perhaps he contracted childbed fever from the woman he autopsied."

"Herr Professor Kolletschka died of childbed fever?"

"I am afraid so, Herr Doctor Semmelweis. I am very sorry."

"Childbed fever?" But no matter how many times in the following days Doctor Semmelweis would ask that question in disbelief, both Semmelweis and his colleagues knew that the horrifying answer was undeniable.

Chapter Nine

Herr Professor Jakob Kolletschka was dead from a cut on his finger. One of those who taught the science of autopsies had himself been killed by a postmortem examination. Jakob was dead of childbirth fever!

A well-liked surgeon and teacher was dead of a nick from a scalpel. He had not been a prostitute whom God had cursed. He had not been a lowly peasant wife divinely punished for her station in life. He was not one of the uneducated and impoverished who were the usual patients of the First Clinic. Jakob Kolletschka had been a professor of forensic medicine, a physician, and a surgeon. And Jakob Kolletschka had died of childbed fever.

The surgeons of the First Clinic were afraid. One of their own, a professor, no less, had now succumbed to childbed fever. No one had previously considered this kind of tragedy. There had been rumors that the English had discovered that the exhalations from women with childbed fever could infect others, but no doctor or midwife had previously contracted the disease. No one had previously imagined that the terrified mothers-to-be could bring about the deaths of their caregivers. Now the English idea was given more credence.

The doctors became very cautious in their movement, whether they were performing a postmortem or examining a mother. They tried not to inhale very deeply around either the mothers and the corpses. Since Doctor Kolletschka had become sick after a scalpel had nicked his finger, doctors now often wore two pairs of gloves. How could that protect them from the deadly exhalations of sick mothers? Logically, it couldn't. But, if childbed fever had thirty or more causes, it seemed prudent to protect against one that had recently proven to be deadly.

"I wear two pairs of gloves during autopsies because it now makes sense," Doctor Rosenberg proclaimed within accidental earshot of his chief resident. "I'm Austrian, not English, so I feel no reason to guard against the noxious exhalations of the corpse I am examining." For days this line produced laughter everywhere it was repeated. Out of respect for their chief resident's loss, the doctors and students made sure that Semmelweis was not in the vicinity when they joked.

The midwives of the Second Clinic were equally frightened. They, too, needed to remain in close company with the mothers-to-be who were admitted to their clinic on non-Death days. Had their patients now been revealed as contagious? Had one more threatening mystery been added to the long history of the vagaries of childbed fever?

Worse for the doctors of the First Clinic, after four months of not being required to do many postmortems, they were now returned to the days before December. Many more autopsies had to be performed. Whether this was caused by a need to explain the death of Professor Kolletschka or simply by the return of Doctor Semmelweis as instructor of autopsies, every surgeon was again expected to perform their quota of postmortems. The doctors were afraid, but committed to their duties.

Doctor Semmelweis watched doctor after doctor return from the ward where the autopsies were performed. They'd stride into the First Clinic and plunge their hands into the genital organs of mothers giving birth. This had always been standard procedure. But Semmelweis had had an epiphany not long after he had read the autopsy report for Professor Kolletschka. The chief resident now had a completely different perspective about the practice of moving directly from the autopsy to the examinations of mothers or mothers-to-be. Previously he had regarded the uterus of an underprivileged woman, like all surgeons, as a filthy place. Therefore, dirty surgeon hands weren't going to have much of an effect.

Moreover, doctors were proud of not being squeamish. It was a badge of honor. The dirtier and bloodier the hands and clothing, the busier the surgeon. Cleanliness indicated a man who was unfit for the surgery profession.

No, Doctor Semmelweis now thought. Wrong. Something had jumped off the autopsy scalpel and had killed his best friend. He was sure of it. He would not yet tell anyone of his suspicion, partly because he knew how crazy his theory sounded and partly because he was now acutely aware of how much of an outsider to Vienna he was. He hadn't forgotten the new note nailed to his office door.

But every instinct told Semmelweis he was right. Something on the autopsy scalpel had killed Professor Kolletschka. Who could deny this? It was the autopsies that were killing the mothers.

It was the autopsies that were killing the mothers!

In England some reputable physicians had been insisting that some mothers-to-be were contagious, that childbed fever was a plague spread from mother to mother. The bad breath of sick m others killed healthy mothers.

That made no sense, Semmelweis knew. The English had missed the true connection between childbed fever and the way it had been spread. Why wouldn't more physicians and midwives have contracted this mothers' fever long ago if all that was required for them to become sick was to breathe the same air as sick women? Why had so many caregivers been immune until now?

Doctor Semmelweis had tried to subtly test the reaction to his theory on two of his medical students, but both had eyed him strangely, as if the death of Professor Kolletschka had unhinged their chief resident. Semmelweis wanted to protest that if the doctors would just examine the data dispassionately, his idea would have much basis. Characteristically, Doctor Semmelweis lost confidence in promoting his hypothesis any further. The fear in both the First Clinic and Second Clinic could not be diminished by logic. And why should reason have prevailed? Nothing had made sense for many years. And now doctors knew they could contract the disease from the autopsies.

Yes, Semmelweis thought. Yes, they could get childbed fever from doing an autopsy. That was correct. That was an obvious conclusion now that Professor Jakob Kolletschka had died from childbed fever. "Let's hope none of these dead mothers breathe on us today," Herr Doctor Meenen had said in morbid jest. No one was yet joking about the material on the scalpel that must certainly be a cause. A nick *in a surgical glove* had allowed this material to fatally infect Professor Kolletschka. Why joke about bad air? The English were wrong. It wasn't contagion that had killed Semmelweis's friend. Why didn't everyone see the simple truth? It was apparent, if one considered the serious sense of the situation, that surgeons did not need to fear each time the corpse exhaled.

Something had jumped off the scalpel into the cut it had made in Professor Kolletschka's finger and had spread disease throughout the doctor's body. This fact was strange. But obvious. It had been childbed fever that had killed Kolletschka or something that had caused the exact same symptoms. No one could deny this terrible development. No one could roll back the weeks to a time before this awful knowledge. Professor Jakob Kolletschka had died of childbed fever contracted from a surgical knife. The autopsy had declared this. The autopsy had proclaimed perhaps the most shocking aspect yet about a disease that defied sane consideration. What a devastating turn of events.

The facts were insane. A previously healthy man of 43 years had died from a minor cut.

Mothers were dying from a traditional contagion, Semmelweis knew. He and his students were not in danger from the air they were breathing. It could not have been the ambient air in the ward where they conducted autopsies that had killed Professor Kolletschka. Something had had to have come off the scalpel used in the autopsy and gone into the cut on Kolletschka's finger.

Semmelweis had tested the contagion theory many times. Women who had been isolated from feverish mothers--women who had never had any apparent contact with sick mothers--still contracted the disease. Even some women who gave birth at home contracted childbed fever, even though the home-birthing mothers had a much lower incidence of the disease. How could childbed fever be caused by a traditional contagion when often there was no evidence of a mother having ever having had previous contact with the disease?
.
No, childbed fever was not a contagion. It was not caused by something in the exhalations of sick women, Semmelweis knew. *It had a cause never before considered in the history of medicine*. Its etiology, its origin, was due to some new reason on which science had never focused. Whatever doctors were searching for, it had been on the blade on the surgical tool. It had been caused by something on the scalpels used in the autopsies. Why then were doctors still insisting it was bad air caused by sick mothers? That was not what the evidence indicated.   Professor Kolletschka had operated outdoors on a woman who was no longer breathing. No. Bad air could not be the cause.

Some kind of particle in the dead mothers was spreading the disease.

Day after day Doctor Semmelweis watched the surgeons go straight from their autopsies and begin examining the mothers who had given birth or who were about to give birth. The hands that probed the mothers' genitals were contaminated by the same unnamed something that had jumped off the scalpel into the blood of his best friend.

Midwives rarely performed autopsies! That was why the Second Clinic had so low a death rate for its patients. Midwives were of course trained by observing and participating in autopsies but certainly at nowhere near the frequency as that of surgeons.

And what had happened during the four months during which fewer and fewer autopsies had been performed? In November 1846 the death rate for mothers had been nearly 11%. But then the number of autopsies had greatly decreased. In December the death rate had been cut in half! In January of 1847 the mortality rate was two-thirds of December, and far less than one-third of November, when the autopsies had been going full steam. By February of 1847 only six women of 312 had died of childbed fever, less than 2% of all women admitted to the First Clinic that month.

It had been the autopsies that had been killing the women. How could Doctor Semmelweis come to any other conclusion? He looked at the statistics for the maternity wards again and again. The waves of childbed fever had reached their zenith exactly during the times when the most autopsies had been performed.

But how could Doctor Semmelweis, the Hungarian outsider, the suspected Liberal, confide his suspicion to Professor Klein? How could he ask for support for his theory from a supervisor who treated him so disrespectfully? And, if he was to confirm his observations, if he was to implement some new procedure to attack childbed fever, he would need the approval of the director of the clinic.

Professor Klein believed in scientific medicine, didn't he? But he also seemed to detest his chief resident. But Professor Klein was a doctor first, was he not? He would not allow his personal feelings to interfere with the health of his patients, would he? But Semmelweis had been forced on the Professor, and Klein had been initially led to believe things about his assistant that were not true. Klein still resented being deceived, even if it had not been by Semmelweis himself.

Doctor Semmelweis wished he could ask Jakob what he should do, but his friend was dead of childbirth fever. To Professor Kolletschka Semmelweis could have spoken of "cadaverous particles" that were transferred from the autopsy tables into the genitals of mothers. Jakob would have listened carefully to Semmelweis's discovery. Jakob would not have summarily rejected the idea. But what about Klein? Would he, as usual, be subjected to the director's ridicule? Did he dare to mention his theory to anyone else?

Yet now everything seemed logical. Now reason was restored. Wouldn't everyone realize immediately that it had to be some particles on the knife that had killed Jakob Kolletschka, and that it was these particles that desperate doctors had wanted to interview for centuries?

But childbed fever had raged for two centuries, for as long as there had been maternity clinics and hospitals for disadvantaged women giving birth. How could Semmelweis suggest that all this time some invisible evil substance had been the cause? It would sound like the ravings of a lunatic, made unstable by the death of his closest friend.

Semmelweis said nothing, but he conducted his own experiment. The chief resident began to cleanse his hands in a cleaning solution of chlorinated lime and water after every autopsy and after every examination of a mother or mother-to-be. Through all of April 1847 the obstetric surgeon waited for his proof. He allowed no other physician to examine his patients.

He was mocked behind his back. Others laughed, "There is a strange new smell in the First Clinic. Oh no, it's just Semmelweis."

But not one of Doctor Semmelweis's patients contracted childbed fever. The chief resident may have been ridiculed, but his results were noted.

Other evidence supported Semmelweis's growing suspicion that tiny particles from the autopsies were the cause of so much disease in the First Clinic. The death rate for the entire First Clinic was over 18% for the month of April, more than a nine-fold jump from February, when very few autopsies had been conducted.

Chapter Ten

Fifty-seven women of the 312 women omitted to the First Clinic in April 1847 lost their lives. Fifty-seven women. But now Doctor Semmelweis thought he finally knew how to prevent these tragedies.

Doctor Semmelweis was more haunted than ever, but how could he go to the professors of Vienna General Hospital and tell them a story about how "cadaverous particles" were killing these mothers?

But how could he not? What is the man who knows the truth and keeps it secret? What is the man who chooses a profession only to ignore his duties and obligations? What is the man who watches terrible suffering and, though he knows he might prevent it, does nothing?

A sham. A lie. A coward.

By the middle of May Doctor Semmelweis could stand it no longer. He requested a meeting with Professsor von Rokitansky.

The Professor was not immediately outraged by Semmelweis's hypothesis. "You believe that your hand-washing is the reason none of your patients have contracted childbed fever?"

"Yes, Herr Professor. I have no proof but..."

"Yes, but... But your theory is unscientific. But your idea is insane. What about the imbalance of humours? Or have you so quickly forgotten your medical training?"

"Our autopsies have always shown very confusing results. We have found no particular organ to stand out as a cause of these fevers."

"What else should you expect? Childbed fever is a very complex disease with perhaps hundreds of factors to be considered and mapped before we can cure it. But chlorine-and-water hand washes? Hand-washing after an autopsy? That seems far too simple a solution to a disease that has so many causes as childbed fever. On the other hand, it might be possible that dirty hands could be a minor factor. We are all shocked by what happened to Herr Professor Kolletschka. It makes no sense to anyone. I would believe just about anything these days."

"He was cut on the finger by a scalpel used in an autopsy. He developed childbed fever. Does that not point conclusively to something on the surgical instrument as a cause of childbed fever?"

"You make an interesting case for your theory. But childbed fever has dozens of causes. How many women do you believe you can save by washing your hands? Do you realize what a simpleton you sound like, Herr Doctor? A lot of women die in the First Clinic. You have not been able to prevent their deaths. You feel like Judas, am I right? If you wash your hands enough times, you will be forgiven and mothers will no longer die? Is that correct?"

"No, Herr Professor, I do not think of myself as a Judas."

"Perhaps as Lady MacBeth, then?" The Professor smiled at his own joke.

"Herr Professor, you taught me to trust my own observations. This last month I washed my hands in a chlorine-and-water solution after every autopsy and before examining any of the women in the clinic. Not one of my patients caught the childbed fever."

"I am trying to stand in your shoes, Herr Doctor Semmelweis. Can you also see things from my point of view? It is impossible for childbed fever to have only one cause. You are being superstitious, Semmelweis. I am not unsympathetic. You have been under a great deal of stress. Your friend, Herr Professor Kolletschka, died. The clinic had almost no deaths for months, and then suddenly right after you return the death rate jumps again. It is an intolerable situation for you. For all of us. But you are grasping at straws. Can't you see that?"

"But disinfecting my hands after an autopsy is, I believe, the reason that none of my patients were sickened last month. While one in five women admitted to the First Clinic contracted the childbed fever."

"That sounds like a coincidence, Herr Doctor. Could not the cause of improvement be Professor Klein's suggestions? That seems much more likely."

"I can see no reason why applying leeches to dying women would greatly increase the numbers of women who do not contract childbed fever. That is not logical."

72

"You're being disrespectful of the director of the First Clinic? Herr Doctor Semmelweis, the bleeding of patients has been an approved technique since the peak of Roman and Greek civilizations. Are you questioning the efficacy of such a proven method?"

Doctor Semmelweis knew when to retreat. "No, of course not, Herr Professor. I am only stating that in the case of healthy mothers, since there is no reason to bleed them or to induce vomiting or evacuation of the bowels, that Herr Professor Klein's recommendations obviously do not apply."

"Perhaps by treating the dying women with Herr Professor Klein's methods, they become less contagious to the healthy mothers."

"Yes, Herr Professor. That seemed like a possibility. But I have isolated healthy mothers from sick mothers upon their admission to the clinic, and yet they have contracted the childbed fever. I do not believe that healthy mothers contract childbed fever from the exhalations of sick mothers. I myself gave these women the disease because I used the same hands to perform an autopsy and to examine mothers giving birth. If we could get childbed fever by breathing the same air as sick mothers, why would not all of us have contracted childbed fever long ago? It is the cadaverous particles that are killing mothers, Herr Professor. I am sure of it.

"Why else would Herr Professor Kolletschka have contracted a disease that is common to mothers giving birth. There was some autopsy material on the scalpel that simultaneously cut into his glove and finger. The particle or particles from the cadaver infected his blood. Herr Professor Kolletschka was a professor of forensic science who had conducted hundreds of autopsies. Why did he only contract a fever when an autopsy scalpel nicked his finger? Over the many years that Herr Professor Kolletschka examined the corpses of childbed fever victims, why did he not become sickened by his contact with them? Why did he only become ill when his blood came in contact with the scalpel used in the autopsy?"

"You are a very clever man, Herr Doctor, a very clever debater. You have thought a great deal about this, Herr Doctor. But to believe that simply disinfecting ones hands after an autopsy will prevent childbed fever seems a very simplistic solution."

"My experiment has so far worked, Herr Professor. I had no dead patients all month. Now I would like to expand my experiment."

"You have shown great diligence, Herr Doctor Semmelweis. And your logic makes a certain kind of sense. It was true that when fewer autopsies were being formed, there were fewer deaths. Unfortunately, one of these deaths was Professor Kolletschka. It is also true that the Second Clinic, whose midwives are seldom at the autopsy tables, have had an impressive success rate since we separated the clinics into surgeons' and midwives' clinics. I have to admit a certain curiosity about these coincidences. I am beginning to wonder myself if some malignant material in dead victims can be one of the minor causes of childbed fever. If you tell anyone that I confessed that to you, Herr Doctor, I will have you committed to the insane asylum. However, you have made a startling argument for your hypothesis. I also know how persistent you will be in pursuing this matter.

"Perhaps we will discover something new with your experiment. However, I cannot have you telling people you believe cadaverous particles are killing mothers, Semmelweis. For your own good. That's not scientific. That's not a reasonable explanation. That sounds crazy."

"Yes, Herr Professor." Semmelweis sensed a weakening of the Professor's reluctance to allow his student to conduct his experiment.

"I hear disappointment in your voice. Professor Kolletschka told me once that your greatest fault was your greatest virtue, Semmelweis. You care too much and do not understand that most people in this world care too little. You offend people by needing to drag them from trivial matters to your own cause. You have that peculiar kind of arrogance, Semmelweis, that springs from your conscience. You are too direct and uncompromising. You cannot wait for other opinions to catch up with you, not while your patients are dying."

Semmelweis didn't know whether he was being rebuked or complimented.

"I believe your only motive is to help your patients. No man who was ambitious or political would act as offensively as you have. And, as I said previously, you have had extraordinary results with your hand-washing innovation, while the rest of the surgeons have amassed a record number of fatalities. We have never before had fifty-seven dead mothers in one month. I am almost inclined to institute your experiment for the entire First Clinic."

Semmelweis tried to phrase his reply so as not to discourage Professor von Rokitansky's surprising reversal. "I believe we would get encouraging results, Herr Professor."

"Herr Professor Semmelweis, I do not believe you understand what a tempest you are about to unleash. You think it is unnecessary to give obeisance to the current state of politics. I fear this character trait will be your undoing. If you institute your innovation, some doctors will resent you even more than they already do. They will not rebel openly against your authority, because you are the chief resident and you are the assistant to the head of the clinic, but they will undermine you in many ways. They will look for ways to rid themselves of you.

"The idea of just 'playing doctor' has never occurred to you? Do you ever consider how you are affecting your possibility of future appointments and honors, Herr Doctor Semmelweis?"

"I'm not sure what 'playing doctor' means. I know I cannot let mothers die without trying to prevent their deaths."

"I think perhaps you may have stumbled upon something that may have a very small role in childbed disease. You are probably giving this hand-washing far too much importance, but perhaps the circumstances surrounding Herr Doctor Kolletschka's accident will actually lead to some bigger discovery. On the hand, more like likely it will turn out to be just a stroke of good fortune that you had no sick patients the month that you kept your hands so clean. Those may have been happy results for the women who left the clinic in a healthy state, no doubt, considering how many departed the First Clinic in a box last month. And, knowing you, Herr Doctor Semmelweis, you are going to attribute your clean hands as their saving grace until you learn the hard way that childbed fever is not a disease that surrenders to simple solutions. Your unexplainable success could turn out to be very unlucky for you, Herr Doctor Semmelweis. Your results last month will probably prove illusory, at the same time that they have encouraged you to take the whole clinic on a wild goose chase.

"Do you understand what you are doing to your career? To your reputation? You are already being mocked by some of the older doctors. Were you aware of this?"

"Yes, Herr Professor. But they are not insubordinate to my face."

"There is a group of doctors even in the First Clinic that would be happy to see you dismissed from your position as chief resident."

"That does not surprise me, Herr Professor."

"No, of course not. They are going to hang you, Semmelweis."

"Who is going to hang me?"

"The doctors who you want to require to cleanse their hands. Do you actually want to ask an Austrian gentleman, someone in his last year of medical school or even a graduate of the University of Vienna, to disinfect his hands before he puts them in the filthy uterus of a Vienna prostitute?"

"Does that seem like such a terrible imposition? Compared to the possibility of saving so many lives?"

"It's an outrageous request, Semmelweis."

"I mean no offense to anyone, Herr Professor. I only want to help these women. Most of these women are not whores. They are just too poor to have a doctor call on them in their own domicile. Moreover, whatever we learn from the mothers of the First Clinic is knowledge that we can apply to the great ladies of Vienna and, perhaps, to all the women of Europe."

"You are sure that the death of your friend has not undone your sense of judgment? It does not occur to you how humiliating it will be for your doctors to pretty themselves up for their operating table dates with the whores of Vienna?"

"I am quite sane, Herr Professor. Even if I am not positive that my conclusions are right. But shouldn't a good scientist have doubts about his own hypotheses, so that his own ego will not lead him to persist on the false path?"

"You've made the right reply, Semmelweis, even if I suspect it may be clever. But tactics in the cause of scientific medicine are admirable. I do not believe your idea will make much of a difference, Semmelweis. But I am curious, also. I also do not think you comprehend how much you are going to be hated if I allow you to go ahead with your hand-washing scheme. You astound me sometimes, Semmelweis. You understand nothing of the world around you. You simply cannot be assimilated into the ways of Lower Austria. Your obsessions are all that you care about. You are an extremely self-absorbed man. You do not care about the traditions and customs of the Empire. You care nothing for the feelings of the medical establishment. You are too obsessed to understand that a Hungarian should not make waves."

"I do not want to offend anyone, Herr Professor. Sincerely, I do not."

"You offend me, Semmelweis. What makes you think that you could solve a mystery that I or Herr Professor Klein or Herr Doctor Skoda have not yet deciphered? You are what, twenty-eight years old? You wanted to be a lawyer. Then you wanted to be an internist. You failed at so much already and yet you think that you can surpass men in the forefront of the medical revolution, three doctors who have more than a half century more experience than you? What arrogance you have."

"I have always had great respect for my teachers, Herr Professor von Rokitansky. I have always admired you and Herr Doctor Skoda. You have taught me everything about the new scientific medicine. I would never intentionally do anything to offend you."

"I should let you go ahead with your experiment, Semmelweis. I am so angry at your rebuttal of my every objection, I should let the doctors of Vienna General Hospital dissect you."

"I would dissect myself if I thought I could have saved mothers but that I had not tried."

"Yes, that's exactly what I thought you would say. You cannot be stopped, Semmelweis. You would find a way around any caution I placed in your path. You are a fanatic. What was it you said earlier about invisibility?"

"That the Lord God is invisible to us, so why shouldn't we regard Satan as an invincible force? I was trying to find an explanation for the cadaverous particles that I believe killed my friend."

"Yes, well don't try to explain cadaverous particles, Semmelweis. Never mention that phrase again. Cadaverous particles. Ask the doctors to wash their hands in your solution after every autopsy. If they examine more than one mother, they are also to cleanse themselves after each examination. Give them no explanation for this request. Never mention cadaverous particles again. It would greatly undermine your credibility and, by extension, mine. This is what you actually believe was responsible for your success rate last month? The washing of hands?"

"Yes, Herr Professor."

"You do understand how much you will be mocked, Semmelweis? The men under your charge are highly-trained surgeons, not five-year-old boys. You will get more resistance from them than from even the most spoiled toddler, and you will have to be constantly watching them, constantly struggling with them. Are you sure you want to do this, Semmelweis? I don't think you understand how much trouble you are going to bring down upon yourself. You could continue as you have done, washing your own hands and recording the results, waiting and washing. You do not have to institute this hand-washing policy right away. You could wait a few months. If you are right about the chlorine-and-water hand-wash, you would not be responsible for the deaths of any mothers under your care."

"But I would be much more responsible for the mothers that died in the First Clinic than anyone else. The surgeons would not know their foul hands had killed the mothers. I would know, though. I would know from what cause the mothers had died. They would have died from the cowardice of Doctor Semmelweis. I would once again be a partner with Death itself. I would in fact have become Death. I would be The Death Of Medicine."

Doctor Semmelweis was afraid he had spoken too vehemently. Would Professor von Rokitansky be even more offended and not grant him permission to begin ordering the surgeons to cleanse their hands? But von Rokitansky sounded only infinitely sad. "I am shocked by the statistics and perhaps a little desperate. I do not believe in your idea, but I am going to let you try it. In a few months you will grow to understand that you have jeopardized your career and your reputation for a fluke. The statistics in The First Clinic are extremely capricious. The death rate will be 20% one month and 2% the next and you will have looked like a fool for having required educated men to cleanse their hands. However, I have no choice but to let you discover your own folly.

"I will not suffer the consequences of my decision, Semmelweis. You will."

"Yes, Herr Professor."

"The director of the First Clinic believes that leeches and emetics and purges were what saved mothers since November. You are his ungrateful and disloyal assistant, Semmelweis."

Semmelweis hesitated, and then gave a reminder that he hoped the Professor would not resent. "Fifty-seven women died last month."

"You will never understand Vienna, Semmelweis." Professor von Rokitansky shook his head sadly. "I thought you had so much promise as a doctor and surgeon, Semmelweis. But I see now that you will never understand Vienna, that you cannot comprehend what I have been hinting to you today. Herr Professor Klein is a good doctor, Semmelweis, but the deaths of fifty-seven poor women will not matter to him even a tenth as much as having been embarrassed by his ungrateful chief resident.

"Herr Professor Klein has been awash in praise for months. He has made an important discovery. He will believe you are trying to rob him of his fame. He will think you are trying to grab his spotlight. If your success continues, he will hate you. Many doctors will hate you. For your sake, Herr Doctor Semmelweis, I might hope that you quickly find that the results of your hand-washing experiment are only a coincidence. I will ask you one last time. Are you sure you do not want to delay asking the surgeons to wash their hands until July or August? There will be many less autopsies in the summer months. You will not inflame so many doctors in the summer."

"If even one more mother died because of me, I would hate myself a hundred times more than Professor Klein ever did."

"Yes, of course. Once again I had expected you to reply in that matter. You will not be stopped, Semmelweis, because you are sure that you are right. I expect that you will now bring a thousand calamities upon yourself and in the process you will not save a single mother.

"And even if by some one-in-a-million chance you have made some tiny insignificant discovery, Professor Klein and his supporters will also not be stopped. Especially if he fears that you are right. I hope you are completely wrong. If you are wrong, perhaps some day your actions will be forgiven."

"I still have your permission, Herr Professor?"

"Of course, you poor damned arrogant soul."

Chapter Eleven

Semmelweis waited until after he had accompanied Professor Klein on his morning rounds before he called a meeting of surgeons. Had Professor von Rokitansky already informed Professor Klein of Semmelweis's plan? He hoped not. Should he have spoken with Professor Klein before he had set out the washing bowls of disinfectant? He had been hesitant to do this. He was apprehensive of the reaction his bowls of disinfectant might receive from the director. Semmelweis finally had decided he would wait to inform the head of the clinic. Professor Klein had always been cool to Semmelweis, since his first day at the clinic. Semmelweis didn't feel he could trust him. Klein would want to rob Semmelweis of any new idea that he sensed Semmelweis felt was important.

Doctor Semmelweis needed to placate Professor Klein. Otherwise the washing bowls would not be allowed to remain in the First Clinic. Baron von Rokitansky was not going to tell Professor Klein what to allow in his own clinic. How could Semmelweis get Klein on his side? The previous evening Doctor Semmelweis had rehearsed ways he would deflect his supervisor's objections to his innovations, if it became necessary. He also planned to pass off his unannounced innovation as a very minor matter, not worthy of the Professor's attention.

As Doctor Semmelweis had promised, he did not speak of cadaverous particles nor give any doctor or student in the First Clinic a reason why they were being asked to clean their hands after autopsies or examinations of the patients. Doctor Semmelweis told the doctors and students he would be relentless, however, in enforcing his new edict.

It happened that Semmelweis did not need to request an audience with Professor Klein. The director of the First Clinic sent for him in the late afternoon. Semmelweis knew from the severe expression on Klein's face that he immediately needed to be very nimble in finding a way around Klein's quiet rage.

"What are these humiliations you are forcing on our surgeons, Semmelweis? I have been receiving complaints all day."

"Humiliations, Herr Professor? I don't know you mean. I am enforcing your suggestions. I believe your ideas are excellent, Herr Professor, and I can't imagine that anyone would object to them. We have had a temporary setback. I do not deny it. The statistics for the last month were the worst the First Clinic has ever suffered, including the death rates during the time of my predecessors. One should not forget, however, that your innovative techniques, which I have strenuously promoted, succeeded miraculously for the previous four months. We only lost six mothers in February. I feel sure, Herr Professor, your improvements toward the treatment of childbed fever will eventually prevail." Doctor Semmelweis was hoping, of course, that from this day forward there would be no sick mothers, in which case he would not have to apply the Professor's ideas. Realistically, he knew he was sacrificing the comfort of some dying mothers in order to protect the living.

Was his supervisor, above all, a dedicated scientist? Did Semmelweis really need to perform this subterfuge which he was almost positive the professor would immediately see through? Not long ago Doctor Semmelweis would have afforded Professor Klein the benefit of the doubt. The Professor was decades the senior of Semmelweis and much more experienced. His snide remarks about the backwardness of Hungary and other locations beyond Austria were not to be excused, but his knowledge of medical technique could not be debated. He could lecture about the various effects of the four humours for hours. His dissection technique was impeccable. His knowledge of human anatomy was supreme. If he was Conservative in political convictions, he was as much a new scientific physician as the Liberals von Rokitansky, Skoda, and von Hebra. Doctor Semmelweis would have preferred to have had Professor Klein as a partner in his experiment, but the innovation was too important to Semmelweis to have it denied by the Professor. Doctor Semmelweis knew that he played a dangerous game in trying to detour the Professor's attention from the hand-washing bowls, but he had become sure he had no other choice.

Doctor Semmelweis had respected the Professor. He and Klein had maintained a coexistence precisely because they both believed in the same medicine and the same curative techniques. Klein knew by now that Semmelweis didn't need to be watched, that he would apply what he had learned at the University of Vienna Medical School, no matter that he was an--ugh!--Hungarian. In return, Klein rarely needed to be consulted by Semmelweis. Doctor Semmelweis had quickly grasped in his first few weeks of residency what his superior expected, what would please him and what would earn his inattention. This relationship had been the best either doctor could expect, since the present circumstances chained them to a daily dance around the other.

Doctor Semmelweis knew it would be risky to change any part of the current

81

tense contract. He must do nothing that would raise the Professor's suspicion, and that included finding a way to make his new hand-washing bowls something the Professor himself had implicitly approved. He must also continue with his flattery of the Professor, even though he was sickened--disgusted--by the treatment he was now praising, although before Jokob Kolletschka's death he himself had found the age-old techniques to be entirely reasonable.

"My improvements?" Doctor Semmelweis had stopped the Professor in his tracks.

"Yes, of course, Herr Professor. The increased application of leeches. The new frequency of enema use. The inducement of vomiting in sick women. I believe we only need to persevere on this path. I have faith in your new treatment, Herr Professor. The other surgeons will soon see that you have found a way to fight childbed fever. They should not feel humiliated because of the changes you have requested. I do not understand why anyone should feel humiliated. In fact I feel that every surgeon in the First Clinic will soon rejoice. You will be a hero of medicine, Herr Professor."

"Oh yes. The changes I suggested."

"I have made it clear to everyone that these improvements belong to you, Herr Professor. I am, above all things, your loyal assistant. I will not accept a drop of credit for all the mothers you have saved. That would be unseemly. That would be wrong. Herr Professor. I feel we must not be discouraged by the tragic numbers of one month! Herr Professor, we cannot go backwards now, just as we were crossing the frontier into a new age for medicine. Herr Professor, I beg of you, do not let some temporarily discouraged doctors dissuade you from a path I know in my heart will lead to great discoveries."

"More leeches? More enemas? More emetics to induce vomiting?"

"Yes, Herr Professor. It worked for four months. Why should anyone plant doubts about your ideas now? It's only envy. We must stay the course, Herr Professor."

"Yes, Semmelweis, perhaps you have a point." Had Semmelweis really convinced Professor Klein that he was now the Professor's great friend and only interested in promoting the Professor's own ideas? Semmelweis had had very little faith that his tactic would work on Professor Klein, who was a very learned man. He hadn't wanted to try to suggest to Professor Klein that the hand-washing bowls had been an improvement he had included in his instructions to Semmelweis. Semmelweis had been skeptical that Klein would fall for such a tactic. Unfortunately, he had been unable to devise a better plan.

Doctor Semmelweis was afraid that at any moment that the Professor would see through his gambit.

"In any campaign there are the first weeks of reluctance, then the weeks of applied insistence, and then the weeks of a formed habit. Herr Professor, it seems as if some are still stuck in the first weeks of reluctance and that is why we have not been completely successful. I have faith that your innovations will prevail, Herr Professor. In the First Clinic we must only overcome the initial reluctance to new ideas."

"Have some doctors rebelled against my program?"

Doctor Semmelweis hesitated a few seconds before answering, as if he had to consider whether to reveal the names of rebel doctors. "The doctors and students in the First Clinic know that I would never tolerate the slightest deviation from the changes you have asked of us, Herr Professor. In the First Clinic they know that I am completely loyal to your ideas. And why shouldn't I be, considering the unprecedented drop in the death rates your recommendations have brought forth? They know I am happy with your program, Herr Professor. They would not try to dissuade me from these changes. They would go a step above me and come to you personally to complain. Of course, they would not attack your ideas directly. They would be devious."

"They would not attack my ideas directly?"

"They would find some minor change in the First Clinic in order to undermine your assistant and thus by proxy, you yourself, Herr Professor." Doctor Semmelweis himself couldn't believe he was daring to be so subtle with his Professor. All his hopes for proving his suspicions that cadaverous particles were killing the poor mothers of Vienna depended, though, on Professor Klein accepting the hand-washing bowls. If Professor Klein told the doctors and student doctors they did not have to submit to such "humiliation", then there was no chance that Semmelweis could institute the change. There would be chance to prove that something like "cadaverous particles" were killing the women. Doctor Semmelweis was banking on diverting Professor Klein's attention from the bowls of chlorinated lime and water and simultaneously, if necessary, presenting the hand-washing bowls as a very small part of Professor Klein's program of improvements.

"These resisters would come to me directly?"

"Yes, of course, Herr Professor. They know I am committed to your recommendations. However, I am, of course, loyal to the director of the First Clinic, and do not want to put any undue pressure upon you. Has there been only one doctor or many doctors complaining about your ideas, Herr Professor? I can, of course, return to the more limited treatments we were applying before I instituted your recommendations of last December. But we had such improvement with the application of your ideas. It seems a shame to me to not allow your innovations more time. But if there are dozens of doctors who believe I am subjecting them to humiliation..."

"Actually just two doctors came to see me this afternoon, Semmelweis."

"You have read the death rate statistics for December, January, and February? Those are the three months after we strictly enforced your innovations." Doctor Semmelweis had already observed that searching for the illusive reasons for the death of so many mothers had created a type of psychological malady he himself had dubbed "loss of belief in logic". Professor Klein and most other doctors were questioning themselves. Semmelweis himself sometimes hadn't been sure that B followed A, or that C followed B, and that something supernatural wasn't one of the causes of disease. There was a susceptibility to confusion among the doctors of Vienna, and occasionally a tendency, as Professor von Rokitansky termed it, to 'grasp at straws'. Doctor Semmelweis was offering Professor Klein a straw, and was using a rush of words to entice him to accept it. He had only the smallest of hope for his deception, and expected at any moment the Professor would put an end to his charade.

"Yes, I have seen the statistics you have been keeping. The drop in the death rate this winter has been truly remarkable."

"I will, of course, revert to the past policy if you ask this of me, Herr Professor."

"No, that will not be necessary."

"I am afraid to undo even the slightest little factor of the program you recommended, Herr Professor. It has done so much to heighten the reputation of the First Clinic."

"Yes, I understand your reluctance to make any unnecessary changes, Herr

Doctor. I do not want you to alter anything. Proceed exactly as you have been doing. I will deal with any complaints. Continue as you have been doing. I merely wanted to hear your progress. You can go now." Professor Klein seemed sincerely convinced.

"Thank you, Herr Professor."

News of the meeting spread throughout the First Clinic. No one had witnessed Doctor Semmelweis's cleverness first hand. The overwhelming impression kept growing that Professor Klein and his chief resident were in absolute agreement. Semmelweis did nothing to discourage this rumor, savoring his victory without confiding in anyone about it.

In the corridors and wards of the First Clinic there were some shocked surgeons. Semmelweis was presumed to be a Liberal, since he was a Hungarian. Professor Klein was an Austrian Conservative.
How could Klein dismiss their complaints against Semmelweis? Certain doctors felt betrayed. They felt chastened a second time. They felt forced into the humiliation of a hand-washing ritual that was completely unnecessary, unprecedented, and unprofessional.

Vienna General Hospital, the behemoth of which the First and Second Clinics were only a part, was dominated by three Liberals: Baron Carl von Rokitansky, a Bohemian whose native language was Czech; the Czech Joseph Skoda, the former Vienna physician for the poor, chief physician of the hospital's department of tuberculosis, and recently appointed by Professor by Baron von Rokitansky against the vehement objections of the rest of the medical faculty; and Ferdinand von Hebra, an Austrian dermatologist of great reputation who had been deeply influenced by the ideas of Baron von Rokitansky. Professor Klein had been the only prominent Conservative in the First Clinic, the only person Conservatives could turn to. Moreover, most of their colleagues in the First Clinic leaned toward either Liberalism or Radicalism.

Now Professor Klein, who also had been influenced by the Baron von Rokitansky's medical revolution and who had agreed for the need for increased autopsies and realistic studies of human anatomy, had sided against the Conservatives in favor of a Hungarian with a ridiculous idea. No wonder some doctors were deeply resentful of the situation. Vienna was their birthplace and now they had to bow and scrape for a Hungarian foreigner in a hospital under the hypnotic suggestion of a Czech Liberal. For some the sword of Damocles seemed poised above their place of employment. At any time the thread of Conservative sense might finally give way and allow the blade of crazy Liberalism to guillotine all of them.

Professor Klein had stabbed his fellow Conservatives in the back. Austrian gentleman had clean hands as a birthright. No Liberal foreigner, no matter what his authority, had the right to ask surgeons to wash their hands.

Who the hell did Semmelweis think he was? This wasn't just Liberal silliness. This was supremely insulting.

To the Conservative doctors, Semmelweis now not only had the blessing of the Liberals Skoda and Rokitansky, but also that of the traitor Klein. Conservative doctors were resentful and they had a God-given right to be angry but they were also terribly chastened. They had expected Klein to be their champion, but he had shocked them.

Semmelweis had won the day. The ridiculous hand-washing bowls stayed.

Semmelweis's cleverness achieved an almost immediate and dramatic result. The poor women of Vienna survived in much larger numbers because of his subtle manipulations.

Chapter Twelve

Doctor Ignaz Semmelweis was either the Devil himself or like Faust, had made some damning deal with Satan. The hand-washing bowls produced immediate and spectacular results, but there was absolutely no scientific reason that they should have. The First Clinic had already been rocked by a succession of insanities, but Semmelweis's innovation was by far the most bizarre. How could this possibly be happening? The surgeons washed their hands in the disinfectant before examining mothers-to-be or mothers giving birth and no one died. But where was the reason? Why? What kind of superstition was this? What did this have to do with the birthing process? Did Semmelweis actually believe there was some cause and effect between clean hands and healthy mothers?

Semmelweis himself believed a new era in medicine had begun. The statistics for the summer only solidified that impression. In June only six mothers died in the First Clinic. In July only three! In August only five. There had previously been periods of time when the death rate had been low in the First Clinic, most auspiciously the period during the winter when the number of autopsies performed had been very low. This time, though, something felt very different. Most doctors felt in the dark and somewhat apprehensive. Something had been discovered from the unexplained success of the previous winter. That was why on virtually every day now Death itself took a vacation.

These were astoundingly low numbers. Professor Klein regarded himself as the cause, and no one dared dissuade him in the least from that delusion. Why shouldn't he hold to this belief? His chief resident himself had earlier convinced Klein that Klein was the agent of the changes.

Everyone else knew that the strange hero was Semmelweis. There was no more insurrection in the clinic, even by those who resented the chief resident. Saint or demon, who was this young, inexperienced doctor and how had he accomplished this? Doctor Semmelweis was untouchable for the moment and more highly regarded now even by those who had doubted him. His hand-washing bowls were having results. To the doctors not prejudiced by their distrust of those not born in Vienna or by the young doctor's previous hesitations, Semmelweis became a god.

Hand-washing bowls were saving these mothers. That was what was occurring before the eyes and hands of trained doctors. It made no sense. Thousands of autopsies had established the truth that childbed fever was an extremely elusive disease. It had many causes. It had not even previously been cured by correcting an imbalance of just one of the four humours. There had been no obvious connection between the disease and some combination of incorrect humor balances. Inducing vomiting and giving repeated enemas to the sick mothers had not reduced the numbers who eventually succumbed to the disease.

But the hand-washing bowls saved mothers. What madness.

Even the world-famous Baron von Rokitansky was shocked. Doctor Semmelweis had taken the death rate statistics to the Professor at the beginning of every month.

The ever-cautious Baron had warned Semmelweis, "You should not talk outside the clinic about these numbers, Herr Doctor. This is probably only some temporary aberration. I have seen this kind of skewing. There may be no science to your innovation, Herr Doctor. There may be no connection between the hand-washing bowls and the diminished numbers of deaths. In addition, there is terrible grumbling about your innovation by some influential Austrian Conservatives and not a little mocking of both you and me. Everywhere your invention is bound to be regarded as mere coincidence. This temporary respite for the poor mothers of Vienna may yet prove to be illusion." Professor von Rokitansky looked his protege in the eyes, trying to find any evidence of rebellion. He still did not believe the chlorine-and-water hand washings could be entirely responsible for the good news from the First Clinic, but most of the young doctors did. He now began to fear the influence of his former student. If Semmelweis was even partially correct, it might be a calamity for the scientific revolution in medicine that the Baron and Doctor Skoda had founded. "You have not spoken of cadaverous particles?"

"I have kept my promise, Herr Professor."

"Hand-washing bowls. I would not be surprised if we were accused of black magic soon. It is not enough that women are not dying, Herr Doctor. Do not delude yourself into believing that you have found a cause for childbed fever. If you begin to elucidate your theory about cadaverous particles, they will begin to pressure me to sanction you. You will not go back on your word?"

"Of course not, Herr Professor." Doctor Semmelweis felt as if he were in the company of the somewhat ignorant Professor Klein and not before the eminent Professor von Rokitansky. Three months of results were not enough? What else but the hand-washing bowls could have saved the mothers? What else but cadaverous particles could have killed his best friend, Jakob?

Professor von Rokitansky was puzzled by the numbers Semmelweis had brought him. The Professor was between a rock and a hard place. He had recommended his student for the post of chief resident because he had been sure Semmelweis would enthusiastically promote his revolution in medicine. He had never expected his protege to stray so far from the path he himself had chopped through the dense jungle of medieval philosophies. He could not, however, abandon the chief resident. That would reflect on his own judgment. He must somehow gradually bring the heedless and obsessed chief resident back to the fold of von Rokitansky orthodoxy. As Semmelweis had been subtle with Klein, von Rokitansky must also be subtle with Semmelweis. The Baron knew how headstrong and stubborn the young doctor could be. "We must wait, Herr Doctor. We must be patient. We must keep observing. You should not stop searching for other culprits. You are still applying the same number of leeches?"

"If the women seem feverish, Herr Professor." In fact, there had been only about a dozen sick women all summer. Previously, in April, the First Clinic had had more than that number of childbed fever cases nearly every week.

What need did the First Clinic have of leeches? Doctor Semmelweis prayed he could soon put the leeches permanently out of work. Professor Klein bragged about how he had increased the bloodletting and the enemas for mothers, though, and Semmelweis wanted the director of the clinic to keep believing his ideas were saving the mothers. Semmelweis must remain clever. For the sake of the poorer mothers of Vienna. For the memory of his best friend, Professor Jakob Kolletschka.

But surely Professor von Rokitansky would have realized that they now rarely needed leeches. Blood-letting was only practiced on women who had contracted a fever, of course. Why would Professor von Rokitansky ask about the leeches? Could Professor von Rokitansky not visualize what was occurring in the First Clinic? Was he just assuring himself that Semmelweis was still pacifying Professor Klein and the other Conservatives?

"You are still following Professor Klein's directives?"

"Yes, Herr Professor." The sufficiently competent and very experienced Professor Klein was a dwarf compared to the giant Professor von Rokitansky.

Yet von Rokitansky seemed to fear Klein. He must be afraid for my sake, Semmelweis thought. I must remain careful. Von Rokitansky's hesitations always made Semmelweis anxious about his own situation, a feeling he didn't have when he was actually in the First Clinic. Most doctors in the clinic trusted Semmelweis.

Now, though, he had the feeling that he no longer had the complete confidence of von Rokitansky. Semmelweis had expected to be congratulated by the Professor he had idolized. Yet Professor von Rokitansky seemed to be trying to discourage Semmelweis. He was attempting to temper Semmelweis. He still appeared to be telling Semmelweis in a polite way that his hand-washing bowls might be as ignorant as believing that vampire bats caused childbed fever.

Doctor Semmelweis was sure sooner or later Professor Klein would discover Semmelweis had tricked him. At that point in time he would only have Professor von Rokitansky to step up and save him and his discovery. He knew that months ago that von Rokitansky would have let him drown. But now that he was succeeding Doctor Semmelweis expected that von Rokitansky would assure his protege that the Professor had his back. Semmelweis knew he badly needed the blessing of von Rokitansky.

"Although it's nearly autumn, the windows are open. You know that 'bad air' has been blamed as a cause of childbed fever for many years?"

How was Semmelweis going to answer this question without sounding insolent? "Yes, Herr Professor, I often consider that factor. I have carefully examined bad air as a cause of childbed fever. But it does not explain why the First Clinic had so many more mothers dying of childbed fever. Six times as many. Seven times as many. Even more sometimes. The First Clinic and the Second Clinic have the same winds wafting through them. They have the same air in winter."

"Have you looked for some difference between the air in the First Clinic and the Second Clinic?"

Madness. Of course Semmelweis had searched for some difference between the two clinics. Again and again. But Semmelweis couldn't protest against this lack of confidence in his diligence. Semmelweis needed Baron von Rokitansky. "I will look into this, Herr Professor."

"Bad air would explain why the summer's statistics are so good. The winds have blown the bad air from the First Clinic." Semmelweis felt horrified.

This seemed like the kind of argument that Klein would make, not Baron von Rokitansky, champion of science and humanism. There were in most years many fewer autopsies in summer, because postmortems were performed most often in the late afternoon when Vienna's heat discouraged even the most hearty surgeon. In addition most medical students vacationed in the summer, and thus there was no need for autopsy instruction to train them in anatomy. Fewer autopsies in summer, fewer cadaverous particles on the hands that touched the mothers in the First Clinic. There was now no longer a mystery why the incidence of childbed fever dropped in the summertime. There were far fewer occasions for cadaverous particles to land on the hands of doctors in the summer months, and even less chance of these cadaverous particles entering the genitals of the women they examined.

But he was not to ever speak of cadaverous particles. Even Doctor Semmelweis saw the sense in this. He scarcely believed in cadaverous particles himself. He had invented the term and the idea because there was nothing else to explain all the abnormalities he had witnessed.

Professor von Rokitansky continued, "I have been told that there are far fewer patients this summer than last. Many doctors believe that overcrowding is what previously caused the high incidence of childbed fever. In June, July, and August of last year the death rates were 13.1%, 18.1%, and 14.4%. You didn't arrive at the First Clinic until July 1st, of course, so I'm not rebuking you in any way for the poor performance of the First Clinic last summer, Semmelweis. I'm merely asking that you compare these numbers with this summer's figures." The previous summer had been an anomaly, but Doctor Semmelweis knew that he could not assert this.

"Yes, Herr Professor."

"The evidence clearly suggests that overcrowding was a major factor in the spread of childbed fever."

The Professor's mind is not functioning logically, Semmelweis thought. Von Rokitansky had the statistics for the First Clinic in front of him. Semmelweis risked a rebuttal of his famous teacher. "But, Herr Professor, we have seen almost exactly the same number of patients both summers."

"What is your point, Semmelweis?" the Baron shouted. "That we are all murderers?"

Doctor Semmelweis was stunned. "I don't know what you mean, Herr Professor. I do not know what people have been telling you. I have never said anything about anyone being a murderer. I would never say such a thing. I have had many of my own patients die. Why would I say such a thing about other doctors? Why would I even think such a thing?"

"We are trying to bring a revolution in medicine to Vienna and the world, Semmelweis. We are scientists now. We do not want to return to the days when the uneducated population could not tell the difference between a barber and a trained surgeon. We do not want to go backward to the time when the bite of a vampire bat explained everything. Science, Semmelweis. Science, not coincidence! Do you understand, Herr Doctor Semmelweis?"

"Yes, of course, Herr Professor."

"You're dismissed, Semmelweis."

From that day Semmelweis was no longer enthusiastic about receiving advice from his former teacher. Instead of rushing to von Rokitansky every month with his reports, he waited until he was summoned. However, this did not happen much after their meeting that day. Semmelweis was seldom invited to the Professor's office.

Chapter Thirteen

Doctor Semmelweis lost confidence in himself and even sometimes in his hand-washing bowls. At times he wondered why he had ever dared to challenge his superiors, albeit ever so gently. Who did he think he was? At other times he felt he was the most brilliant of all surgeons at Vienna General Hospital. His superior, Professor Klein, was an idiot. His students were idiots. Even von Rokitansky was an idiot. Semmelweis had lost a good deal of respect for his profession. He thought many doctors only played at a subtle game. The main goal was not to find cures but to become champion eventually. To be king of the hill in a game without principle.

Semmelweis still cared for the fate of his patients. They would never be a means to an end for Semmelweis. Their health itself was the goal. Every day. They would never be pieces on a chessboard. But the line between being someone "playing doctor"-- the term von Rokitansky had once introduced to him--and being a good chief resident was now blurred. Semmelweis was being drawn into the meaningless conflict at Vienna General Hospital. He guessed that Professor von Rokitansky was being pressured and compromised and this suspicion cowled him. If the Professor renowned throughout Europe could not defend science, if he refused to admit the conclusions of Semmelweis's simple observations, how could Semmelweis himself be so bold as to insist that hand-washing bowls were saving lives?

Doctor Ignaz Semmelweis was now being forced to consider matters far outside of surgery in order to continue being a surgeon. He needed to play a dozen simultaneous games of chess against opponents with clever strategies.

Semmelweis was disillusioned. What difference was there between the pedestrian Klein and the von Rokitanskys, Skodas, and von Hebras that everyone praised? Liberals versus Conservatives? Let both their houses be damned for eternity. Did any of his superiors feel any great need to quiet the screams of dying women? Wasn't the "scientific revolution in medicine" espoused by von Rokitansky, Skoda, and von Hebra just a dazzling sham? How had it ever saved anyone? What distinguished this new medicine from the medicine of medieval barbers if doctors must ignore the evidence before their own eyes? What was so progressive about this "unprecedented advance"? What diseases had been solved?

Semmelweis felt alone, alternately superior and inferior. He had had a revelation in the office of von Rokitansky. Medicine was presently, and perhaps had always been, about playing a well-defined role. Helping patients was only secondary, maybe even tertiary, to the real goal of "science". The sick mothers of Vienna would have been better off without doctors. On the other hand, doctors needed sick mothers or they could not call themselves surgeons. One could not compete over tea with other physicians otherwise, nor impress the wealthier young women and matrons of Vienna.

But how could he, Semmelweis, challenge the prevailing medical climate? He was a nobody. What had he himself done that was so important? Who was he compared to Skoda or Klein or von Rokitansky? These men had great reputations, while Semmelweis was despised. Semmelweis had thought his superiors would support him, and that the force of their influence would have promoted the hand-washing bowls that were saving so many lives. That wasn't going to happen! Doctor Semmelweis was alone. He no longer had the support of his teachers, a situation he had never anticipated.

Doctor Semmelweis needed some great achievement or he would be doomed even in his own eyes. He also needed some shield to protect him from those who wanted only the most minor excuse to damn him.

He was already twice cursed, He was a Hungarian, and he was thought of as a Liberal in Conservative Austria. He had only remained above water because he was a medical school graduate of the prestigious University of Vienna. His medical degree and profession were all that kept him afloat on a lonely sea.

Semmelweis became even more cautious. He became doubtful of his previous convictions. Maybe Professor von Rokitansky was right. Maybe Semmelweis shouldn't make waves. He would be an object of pity and ridicule if he wasn't reappointed to his current position. He needed the great achievement of being the chief resident of a maternity clinic at the renowned Vienna General Hospital, or else he would be a pariah. Otherwise he would be a dismissed chief resident in addition to being a Hungarian and a presumed Liberal.

Maybe Professor von Rokitansky was right. He had created three strikes not only for himself, but for the great man who had recommended Semmelweis for the position of chief resident. What a clueless ingrate he was being, Semmelweis thought.

Hand-washing bowls? Doctor Semmelweis was asking doctors and medical students nearing the end of their training to wash their hands? He deserved to be mocked and hated, Semmelweis sometimes believed. What had he been thinking? He had wrecked his own career and possibly severely damaged those of Baron von Rokitansky and Doctor Skoda.

Did the doctors at the First Clinic sense his new vulnerability? But Semmelweis saw no visible signs of rebellion among the doctors and medical students of the First Clinic. Occasionally he observed someone arriving from the autopsy room, and giving their hands only a peremptory scrubbing. He'd look away and say nothing.

In the autumn and early winter of 1847 the death rate in the First Clinic doubled. Semmelweis thought it might be because he had lessened his grip, that other doctors sensed he was afraid to insist on hand-washing.

The statistics were still much better than they had been before Semmelweis had set out the bowls of disinfectant in mid-May. Less than four dozen mothers died between the beginning of September and the end of 1847, still far fewer than in the entire month of April. Yet the temporary uptick in the number of mothers who contracted a fatal fever after childbirth led credence to the belief that the disease itself was capricious. It came and went, and no logic could predict its waxing and waning. Death rate statistics, according to this point of view, were bound to rise and fall on their own. Doctor Semmelweis had hurt the case for a connection between "autopsy hands" and childbed fever by not enforcing his own edict.

But if Semmelweis was now timid in his enforcement of his own edict--could something as simple as hand-washing truly save so many lives?--shouldn't the death rates have returned to their previous high levels?

No. The hand-washing bowls were now a fixture in the clinic. Many doctors still used them. As Semmelweis himself had once predicted, the weeks of reluctance and the weeks of applied insistence had now become the weeks of a formed habit. The unexplained drop in the number of mothers sick with childbed fever had eventually brought many doctors in the First Clinic to the same conclusion that Doctor Semmelweis himself had had following the death of his best friend, Professor Kolletschka. The doctors had changed nothing in their daily routine except the hand-washings. Yet there had been a dramatic difference in the number of mothers who stayed healthy after giving birth. That was enough to convince many doctors that the hand-washing ritual was useful.

Some medical students disdained using the disinfecting bowls, but most students began to believe in them. Semmelweis was either unaware of this faith in his invention, or skeptical of its staying power. His students believed in him, despite the deliberate distance Semmelweis maintained between medical students and chief resident.

Semmelweis had been stung by the notes on his office door, by the unpredictability of Professor Klein, and by the unexpected outburst from Baron von Rokitansky, and had become somewhat paranoid. He was not discussing why he had chosen to introduce hand-washing bowls--what sane man, as assailed on all sides as Semmelweis was, would speak of murderous "cadaverous particles" jumping from a scalpel blade to the blood of a human. This sounded even less probable as an explanation than vampire bites. Semmelweis would be damned if he spoke of his strange theory, but would soon be damned because he hadn't.

But, if Semmelweis was afraid of speak of the ablutions of the hands, the young doctors and medical students of the First Clinic were not. Unexpectedly, Semmelweis's hand washing edict became the subject of conversation everywhere. His hand-washing bowls, to Semmelweis's amazement, were soon being discussed throughout Europe, and even in Great Britain.

Semmelweis's students had spread the news of the drastic reduction in death rates at the First Clinic. Their teacher had as yet provided no scientific explanation for the effectiveness of the new medical technique, but it was sufficient for them to trumpet the dramatic statistics. There seemed to be a good deal of evidence for a mysterious link between the autopsies performed and the incidence of childbed fever. Semmelweis had demonstrated that by citing the low mortality rates when and where few autopsies had been done, and this startling connection was debated everywhere. Most notably, there had been a remarkable drop in deaths during the winter of 1847 when public health officials and Baron von Rokitansky hadn't pressed for autopsies. There had also been the unexplainable gap between First and Second Clinics in fatal childbed fevers since 1841, when the clinics had been separated into distinct domains for doctors and midwives. Finally, there was the astounding difference that the washing of hands after an autopsy had made.

In April of 1847 fifty-seven women had died of childbed fever in the First Clinic. Doctor Semmelweis had set out the hand-washing bowls in the middle of May. From June through the end of the year, only once had as many as a dozen women died in the clinic in a month. In another month only three women had succumbed to childbed fever. Even the autumn's temporary uptick, for which Doctor Semmelweis later found a logical explanation, resulted in rates far better than past history. In the long chronology of the disease Semmelweis's results were unprecedented. Who needed a scientific explanation? Someone could add that later, students had thought, after the medical world became aware of Doctor Semmelweis's new innovation in the care of mothers.

Letters from Semmelweis's students were sent to the directors of prominent maternity clinics in Europe.

So bits and pieces of Semmelweis's idea were propagated. The dissemination of Semmelweis's innovation proceeded like a game of "telephone". One person in Europe whispered in another's ear, "Ignaz set out hand-washing bowls", and another whispered the secret, and then another. A thousand whispers later the cure emerged as, "Ignaz believes isolating the women is the goal". Semmelweis's ideas and proofs became mangled because Semmelweis and others believed it wasn't yet prudent to publish his results. For decades there would be misconceptions about what Doctor Semmelweis was advocating. For instance, in England, doctors were told that Semmelweis had proved that sick mothers were the cause of the disease. The English were glad that someone in ignorant Austria had finally caught up with English medicine. They had long espoused contagion as the main cause of childbed fever.

This is exactly what Oliver Wendell Holmes had said in 1843, that childbed fever is contagious, that mothers with the fever could infect other mothers. Was the Austrian medical community so backward, so far behind the advances of the English? Had the chief resident of the maternity clinic at the most advanced hospital in Europe not read of Holmes' theory? That seemed inconceivable. More likely, Semmelweis was trying to steal credit from Holmes.

Actually, Semmelweis had said nothing. He had written nothing. He had published nothing.

How could he? Semmelweis finally had realized how tentative his position had become.

Most surprising to Semmelweis, Ferdinand von Hebra, a follower of Baron von Rokitansky, founder of the New Vienna School of Dermatology, first described Semmelweis's results in December, 1847, and then again three months later. Von Hebra was the editor of a prominent Austrian medical journal. He compared Semmelweis's innovation as equal in greatness to that of Edward Jenner, who had introduced cowpox injections to vaccinate against smallpox.

Doctor Semmelweis stayed silent. He could no longer gauge the atmosphere at the First Clinic and beyond. He didn't think he could depend on anyone for any but the most shallow support. The powers-that-be in Austrian medical circles wanted to hear from Semmelweis himself, but he was extremely reluctant to do so. Since the outburst from Baron von Rokitansky, he was far too fearful and distrustful of the sea in which he swam.

There are eras in human history when true progress becomes immersed in a thick cloud propelled by a strong and capricious wind. A great fog collapses around a major invention as it is moved toward the horizon. It can be seen only dimly until it eventually disappears from view. The late 1840's were such a time. Semmelweis saw his amazing successes, even when they were correctly reported, reduced to one dust particle in the cloud, just as valid in the flow of ideas as increased usage of leeches or any other technique.

He had expected Doctor Skoda and Baron von Rokitansky, the two founders of the Modern Medical School of Vienna, to have been energized by his discovery of the connection between autopsies and childbed fever. Neither doctor immediately stepped forward as his champion. Instead, he and his ideas seemed to have been dismissed, or worse, regarded as dangerous impolitic coincidences.

Was the Modern Medical School of Vienna only concerned because Semmelweis's statistics seemed to accuse the flood of autopsies Baron von Rokitansky had encouraged in the name of science? Was this the meaning of Baron von Rokitansky's strange rebuke? Semmelweis himself had performed many autopsies and then gone directly to assist mothers in a difficult labor or to examine those who had just given birth. He was deeply troubled by his own discovery. If there were something like the "cadaverous particles" Semmelweis theorized, then they had undoubtedly been on his own hands as well. He would have been as much a "murderer" as von Rokitansky. Surely the Baron must realize this. If Semmelweis judged what surgeons had previously done in ignorance, he must condemn his own soul also.

But none of them should ignore the results of the present to hide the mistakes of the past. Yet Semmelweis himself seemed to have chosen this path. He seemed aloof to physicians intrigued by his results in dramatically lowering the death rate in the First Clinic. His link between autopsies and childbed fever made sense, but Semmelweis did nothing to promote his points. Many thought he must be hiding some secret, a deception, or that he was arrogant. Semmelweis was simply unsure of himself. He saw pools of quicksand everywhere and was afraid to take a step.

Doctor Semmelweis now conceded that Baron von Rokitansky had had a point. If autopsies were blamed everywhere as the cause of childbed fever, then Baron von Rokitansky, the scientific revolution in medicine, the study of anatomy, and even the influence of Liberalism in general would probably be burned at the stake. Stupid Semmelweis. What great evil had he brought down on Europe?

Yes, Doctor von Hebra proclaimed his results, but couldn't he just as quickly some day denounce Semmelweis and his statistics? Semmelweis was in charge of noting the fatalities in his own clinic. The numbers that were being shown around Europe were unbelievable to many physicians. There was no independent verification of Semmelweis's results, and seemingly little interest in conducting such science. It would be easy to claim that Semmelweis was greatly exaggerating his success. It would be beneficial to all doctors, Liberal or Conservative, to regard Semmelweis as a liar. As it was even easier during the present time to yawn.

The chief resident at Vienna General Hospital's First Clinic has greatly reduced the mortality rate for childbed fever. Hmmm. That's interesting.

Perhaps. Maybe. Let's think about it. Let's wait and see. Word got back to the chief resident about the indifference elsewhere. On one day Semmelweis would think, damn them. Why aren't they trying to replicate my results in their own clinic? On alternate days he might think: It is good they are not yet making too much of my death-rate statistics. It is good there is some publicity for my numbers but not too much. I am safer if my statistics are not being discussed too much.

Moreover, was there interest in Semmelweis's hand-washing bowls only because the political climate? Von Hebra was a Liberal. Most of Semmelweis's students were Liberals. Semmelweis, because he was Hungarian, was assumed to be a Liberal. He had been graduated from the University of Vienna medical school, a hotbed of Liberalism. Medical students were already leading the charge against the Conservative status quo. Was there support for Semmelweis's innovation only for his assumed politics? Was Semmelweis in the process of becoming a political playing piece? Semmelweis didn't want his innovation sullied by a Liberal versus Conservative dichotomy. He was a scientist. He wanted a discussion with other scientists.

Yet, no matter how little he spoke about his hand-washing bowls, the spotlight was upon Semmelweis. He could not silently hide the monthly numbers without being suspected of having always fudged them. He had to go forward. Other doctors were now watching the First Clinic more closely. In 1848 Semmelweis would be forced to enforce his hand-washing protocol very strictly. He was now forced to prove that he was not a liar, and that his innovation was not nonsense. Or lose reputation and credibility.

Because the reluctant Doctor Semmelweis was forced to stay on the straight and narrow path he had started upon with his hand-washing bowls, his requirements were again enforced. It was less of a struggle this time. His hand washing technique had become more and more justified in the eyes of many in the First Clinic and beyond.

During the entire year of 1848, deaths from childbed fever virtually disappeared from the First Clinic.

Chapter Fourteen

In February of 1848 only 2 mothers died of childbed fever; in March, none! It seems as if this continuing success in Vienna should have brought bowls of disinfectant wash to every maternity clinic in the civilized world. Nothing close to that scenario happened.

Was it because the year was 1848, one of the most fateful years in world history? Was it because political turmoil was everywhere, in France, in Italy, in Poland, in Germany, in Hungary, and, yes, in Vienna?

Would supportive investigations have been given to Doctor Semmelweis's correlation between "autopsy hands" and death by childbed fever if he had been in America or England, and not in Austria? Would a whole new area of medicine have opened if the startling low death rate statistics of the First Clinic in the latter half of 1847 and the entire year of 1848 had not been circulated in an "us-versus-them" era and place?

It seems probable. Semmelweis was distrusted and disbelieved, often because his discovery was both a terrible stroke to the personal self-esteem of both Conservative and Liberal physicians and to their public standing as well. It was only natural for many doctors to congratulate him on his results and at the same time fervently wish for the miracle in the First Clinic to be due to something other than the surgeons' own faulty techniques. And, if a reversal of the link between doctors and the decades of death didn't soon occur, Vienna General Hospital needed some great fogging event that would push Semmelweis's embarrassing new prominence into the background, something that would blur the chief resident from the view of all but those closest to him. Outside of some of his students and, strangely, the prominent Liberal dermatologist Professor von Hebra, no one promoted Semmelweis's discovery, no one disseminated his statistics, no one trumpeted his triumph over a two-centuries-old scourge. Semmelweis's simple idea had worked, but saving the lives of poor mothers had a very low priority.

The great obscuring cloud for which so many had unconsciously or consciously wished had long been on the horizon. The previous few years had seen crop failure, recession, food shortages, drops in the standard of living, and resentment of suppression of so many rights by the Conservative Habsburg regime. Some people called the governing force of the time a "liberal monarchy" with royalty (the Emperor, or "Kaiser") accompanied by elected "Diets" (similar to Congresses or Parliaments). Only the most wealthy males, however, were allowed to vote. The European governments of 1848 had only nominal resemblances to the radical "popular democracy" formed on the American continent in the 1780's. The United States, moreover, had no King or Emperor, no "divine right of kings", no political dynasties on which people could rely for stability in times of change. American-style "Radical" government was not something that the vast majority of Europeans wanted. They feared such independence.

The kind of revolution seen on the American continent had had its counterpart in Europe in France. France, in fact, had been America's staunchest ally in the 1780's. However, the French revolution had taken a completely different course than the American upheaval. The English writer Charles Dickens would outline the common disgust with the French struggle in his "A Tale of Two Cities" (1859). Moreover, after 1815 and the final defeat of Napoleon, there was a reaction against the excesses that had blown from France to seed themselves in other parts of Europe.

A suppression of constitutional liberties, national minorities, and Liberalism had followed. The revulsion toward the previous era led to the restoration of kings, ruling families, and the traditional Conservative authorities of the past.

However, like the French proverb "the more things change, the more they stay the same", the year 1848 had repeated the same conflicts and desires of two and three generations earlier. This return to the uncompromising political pressures and fissures of the early part of the century not only doomed many participants in the succeeding drama, but also condemned mothers throughout the world who otherwise might have been delivered from the agony of childbed fever. The politics of the era became the shoulder-height muck through which Semmelweis and his student supporters struggled to advance.

And where did this new cycle of presumably-already-resolved grievances and counter-reactions begin? In France, of course. There King Louis Phillipe relieved his unpopular Prime Minister on March 23rd in response to demonstrations against the "liberal monarchy". A day later the king himself abdicated.

These events might previously have not been known for quite some time outside of Paris. And, of course, by the time the news had reached other parts of Europe, who knows what could have happened in the meantime? Perhaps all the issues of the struggle had already been resolved. Distant occurrences in the eighteenth century were like light from a star. Who knew if the source of what had been sent was still in existence?

However, now in the middle of the nineteenth century there was the telegraph. It played an underestimated role in the conflicts to come. The telegraph transmitted news of a victory against Conservative suppression in France. In cities throughout Europe Liberals felt that the triumph in Paris could be duplicated in their own cities.

This affected both Semmelweis's native country and his adopted country. The Emperor of Austria held a dual title as King of Hungary. The most prominent Hungarian Liberal, while assuring Vienna that he had no wish to challenge this arrangement, indicated that the Habsburg (Austrian) Empire needed to allow much more independence to the Kingdom of Hungary. The "union enforced by bayonets" should become a "free constitution" alliance for all the nationalities. Since the Magyars (Hungarians) were less than a half of the population of the Kingdom of Hungary, the Hungarian Liberals had to be careful to associate with themselves the interests of the smaller minorities of Hungary, so as not to frighten them into agreements with Habsburg interests. The Empire, on the other hand, needed these minorities as allies in order to counter the Hungarian threat.

Nearly at the same time as their Magyar Hungarian allies, the university students of Vienna marched by the thousands on March 13th, demanding reforms. Soldiers from the Austrian military fired into the crowd, killing some of the demonstrators. This turned the current of opinion against the Austrian royal family and its troops. Prince Metternich, who for so long had been the glue holding the disparate areas of the Austrian Empire together, who was both hated and feared by the Liberals, resigned and fled into exile. The Austrian military, chastised for shooting unarmed Austrian demonstrators, deferred to the Citizen Guard, many of whom were also seeking Liberal reforms. The Guard began to issue arms to many of the demonstrators.

Who was one of the leaders of the Vienna demonstrators? None other than the half-Hungarian writer, politician, and Vienna General Hospital physician Adolf Fischhof. Semmelweis was now not only a member of a minority at war with the Habsburgs and European Conservatives, he was also a member of a politically suspicious profession. Medical students and faculty were complicit in the opposition to the authoritarianism of Conservative rule. They demanded from the monarchy the kind of civil rights already accepted in constitutional democracies, such as freedom of the press and trial by jury. In addition, the faction lead by Fischhof asked for more rights for minorities and a federalist type of system for the non-Austrian territories. Fischhof, still loyal to the idea of a Habsburg constitutional monarchy, felt that without reforms the Habsburg Empire would eventually fragment into nationalities and their fiefdoms. Fischhof also feared the German Liberals who led Liberals of all nationalities would eventually dominate all minorities in the Habsburg Empire. Hungarians, Poles, Slavs, Italians, French, Romanians and many others would be second-class citizens under German rule. Even the freedoms they had enjoyed under Habsburg rule would be lost if German Liberals won the day. Adolf Fischhof was later seen as incredibly prescient.

The Austrian Emperor seemed to quickly concede to the demands of the demonstrators, announcing on March 15th that non-Hungarian parts of the Austrian Empire (sometimes referred to as "Lower Austria") would have a constitutional convention with delegates drawn from all Lower Austrian geographical entities.

A few days after the demonstrations had begun in Vienna, on the Ides of March 1848, Radicals in the emboldened Hungarian Kingdom demanded independence. The Radicals would no longer settle for coexistence with Habsburg rule. This was a turning point in the history of the Habsburg Empire. It could even be argued that it was a watershed moment in the history of Europe, an event that would change the dynamic so drastically as to have consequences for more than a century. The Austrian-Hungarian marriage appeared headed for a nasty divorce, encouraging many other brides of the Emperor to dare to ask for more liberty or even to sue for dissolution. Austrian Conservatives knew that Hungarian aspirations had to be quickly defeated in a manner emphatic enough to discourage other minorities from being disloyal to the Austrian Empire.

The Liberal and Radical outbreaks were spreading to many other parts of the Empire. Many of the German states began to add Liberal provisions to their previously limited Constitutions, or creating first-ever constitutions for their states. Karl Marx published his famous book "The Communist Manifesto", creating a new and unexpected threat to the Austrian Empire and Emperor. A secessionist Europe seemed about to break into many pieces.

In the years preceding 1848 there had been no major movements against the Emperor. All the squabbles were in the family. There had been some violence, seemingly regretted terribly each time by the authorities. "My God, I've hurt my own brother," was the apparent reaction each time his military forces had acted. In 1848 the atmosphere was much more dangerous. Political disagreements and territorial demands didn't just flare for a week or so and then subside. The Austrian Conservatives, caretakers of order in the Empire, didn't just settle for a warning reaction followed by a quick retreat to previous positions. 1848 became the year of all-out warfare.

But during the first seven months of the year the reluctance of the Austrian Emperor to take harsh enough measures led to a seemingly permanent victory for Liberals in many parts of the Empire.

In Prussia the King seemed the only breakwater against the rising waves of Liberalism. He declared that no force could compel him to "transform the natural relationship between prince and people" into a constitutional arrangement. However, he was soon forced into an about-face.

In Berlin, the capital city of the powerful Kingdom of Prussia, which was directly north of and bordered on the Austrian Empire, soldiers fired on and slew nearly 200 demonstrators. As in Vienna, the rulers of Berlin seemed chastened by the massacre and quickly promised concessions. By March 31st preparations were being made for an election.

But in Vienna in April the new constitution satisfied no one. Conservatives resented the seeming weakness of the Emperor's stance. Liberals claimed the new constitution still allowed the right to vote only to the most wealthy men and even with two legislative houses still reserved most of the power to the royal family. The new constitution was a clever trick, they said. The demonstrators returned to the street in earnest.

In May the Austrian Emperor fled Vienna for Innsbruck. For most Austrians of any political allegiance it must have seemed like the beginning of the end for the Habsburg Empire. How could Austria possibly control so many challenges?

In mid-May Conservative forces, sickened by the flight of the Emperor, moved to deny freedom of assembly for the students. Again soldiers fired into the crowds of demonstrators. Again the students were supported by the Citizen Guard and thousands of working class citizens. The protests intensified. The government of Vienna became fearful and compromised, promising to provide jobs, to increase wages and reduce hours for workers, to allow more freedom of speech, and to force landlords to lower their rents.

On June 22nd the new legislative gathering eased tensions. The terrible fog began to clear, the political storm calmed, and the traditional rewards for such stability were paid. There were more jobs. New rights were promised.

The Austrian Emperor returned to Vienna. For the time being there was peace.

Throughout all of this turmoil why would hand-washing bowls and the health of poor mothers accrue much attention? Moreover, beyond the First Clinic, Doctor Semmelweis still did not have much standing. Incredibly, his successes impressed practically no one.

In addition to his other reasons for keeping a low profile, Semmelweis now feared for his family in Hungary, where his brothers were suspected of being involved in the Hungarian independence movement. Doctor Semmelweis retained the hand-washing bowls in the First Clinic, but he spoke to no one of his reasons for having the doctors wash their hands, Some of his students and even Professor von Hebra had hailed his achievement, but Semmelweis had said nothing.

"I feel completely frustrated by the medical establishment," he told his students, Eckhof and Rosenberg. He had realized he could not keep the sympathies of his students unless he confided to some of them more often. He missed the council and friendship of Jakob Kolletschka.

"You should publish," Rosenberg insisted. "You should tell your own story."

"This is not yet a good time. I will be attacked. I know I will be viciously attacked."

"Then wait. The Emperor has given in to the Liberals. There will be a Liberal constitutional government soon. The Liberals will be in control soon."

Yes, but exactly what was a Liberal? Most Austrians and some nationalist movements still did not challenge the idea of a constitutional monarchy. They were loyal to the Habsburg Emperor. They wanted a parliament or congress of Liberals within the framework of the monarchy. But the definition of Liberal depended on which geographical location, economic class, or minority a person represented. Semmelweis had many strikes against him, something his Austrian Liberal friends didn't seem to realize. Despite their participation in the demonstrations, and true to the climate of the time, the Austrian medical students and doctors remained part of the mainstream. Semmelweis, on the other hand, had never felt more isolated. The famous Bohemian Czechs of Vienna General Hospital, Semmelweis's benefactors, Baron von Rokitansky and Doctor Skoda, were supporters of the constitutional monarchy. They were Liberals who only wanted certain reforms. Hungarians, on the other hand, had declared independence! Hungarians were Radicals, animals who wanted the disintegration of the Austrian Empire. Hungarians wanted chaos.

By the middle of the summer the Conservatives had conceded to many Liberal demands. Freedom of the press and other democratic liberties became a reality. There were new parliaments that held elections. But the citizens were afraid and confused, and chose people with whom they were already familiar. The wave of elected Liberals were, in many instances, the former Conservatives. Instead of stabilizing Vienna and other areas, the new governments led to more demonstrations and to fragmentation. In the Austrian Congress there was a Polish faction, a German faction, a Czech faction, and so on, and within each of these nationalist groups were other large fragments. The so-called stability seemed fragile. No one seemed to understand what lasting changes the Liberal victories represented.

Austrian Liberal medical students celebrated a bright new humanist future, but Doctor Semmelweis foresaw the accumulations of the previous storms as an forming the basis for an inevitable avalanche. This was a major reason Semmelweis still wrote nothing, published nothing, and gave speeches nowhere. There was a war, and for Liberals and Conservatives both, he was associated with a dangerous nationality. He could count on no one for support. Moreover, he still could not give a "scientific" reason for forcing surgeons in the First Clinic to disinfect their hands after an autopsy. He had only the suspect statistics. Semmelweis, who had once considered being a lawyer, knew that many doctors would claim he still had only "circumstantial" evidence of a cure.

Chapter Fifteen

One of Doctor Semmelweis's brothers was fond of saying, "Human speech must be either logical, political, inconsequential, or non sequitur, and no category of discourse ever infects the other in the slightest." The profession of medicine was presumed to be dedicated to logic, and thus occupied a category outside the political arena. As apprehensive as Semmelweis was of his status as a Hungarian in Lower (non-Hungarian) Austria, he also felt somewhat protected by his environment. He was among gentlemen, whatever their politics. He and they usually spoke only of the condition of his patients and the progress of their treatments. The turmoil in the streets of Vienna and the other cities of Europe was a world distinct from Vienna General Hospital, never to be transgressed by either demonstrators or soldiers.

Occasionally Semmelweis would overhear some of his students discussing the events in the city itself and, though he did not want to seem to be spying on them, he also wanted to understand their passion. He wanted to feel that their emotions were sincere so that he could address them directly with the doubts in his mind. All of the events in Vienna puzzled him. The protests seemed illogical not because of the demands, which would have been natural concerns for citizens who were hungry, unemployed, silenced, fearful of ever improving their status in lives, or any combination of these disadvantages. But the demonstrations in Vienna had been led by highly educated medical students and Professors. The peasants and lower classes led difficult lives. But why should these students and doctors care? He wanted to believe that their motives were compassionate, but he was also afraid that their commitment to their ideas was weak, fashionable, and fleeting.

"It is like a badly-written tragedy that repeats the same act over and over," Rosenberg told Eckhof one afternoon. "In every city the Liberals demonstrate. The soldiers rush in and fire into the crowd, and then they run back to their sanctuaries. The Emperor or the King feels horror at the loss of life and promises changes. Weeks pass by, and the Conservatives begin to reconsider. They retract their pledges. The students and workers take to the streets again, and they repeat the First Act..."

"At least the Emperor expresses regret, my friend. At least the revolution remains a family affair. I have heard that Jellachic has gathered 50,000 soldiers to protect the Emperor's throne and will march on Hungary soon if they do not forget their demands for independence. General Radetsky has an equally strong army to quell the rebellions on the Italian peninsula. We should be relieved that the Generals do not march in Vienna itself."

"The Hungarians have no respect for the Austrian Emperor's authority. The Austrian Emperor is their King, but they give only lip service to his rule. They deserve to be disciplined."

"The Emperor is weak and the Hungarians sense it. Lower Austria should appease the Hungarians with reforms, as long as the Magyar Hungarians pledge loyalty to the Emperor."

"The Magyars are ruining everything, my friend. They are no longer asking for reforms. They want to get rid of the Emperor. They are part of Austria and they want to do away with the Emperor. The Austrian Emperor cannot be reasonable when the Hungarian Radicals are making such demands. He is forced to crush the Radicals. The Hungarians are forcing the Emperor to crush Liberalism. Because this Hungarian radical Liberalism is becoming too much of a threat to stability. We will lose everything we have gained. There will be chaos. The Hungarians will force a reaction that will doom Liberalism everywhere, even here in Vienna."

"Quite the opposite. The Hungarians will be our strength. The Hungarians are the most warlike people in Europe. Our Emperor does not want a conflict. The Hungarians could easily defeat Jellachic. The Emperor realizes this and he will cave in to Liberal demands The Hungarians will be our threatening sword. The Hungarians will force Austria to become more humanist."

'I don't think so, my friend. Everywhere but Hungary the people want Liberal reforms. They do not want the end of Habsburg rule, only Habsburg reasonableness. The Hungarians will frighten everyone and drive them toward the Conservative cause. The Hungarians have gone too far in their demands. It will be the ruin of all of us."

"No, a new Age of Liberalism is dawning. It's the inevitable progress of history. The Liberal triumph has been long in coming. We cannot lose. The new liberty is inevitable. There will soon be justice for all nationalities and for all classes."

Semmelweis had attended the University of Vienna and recognized the same kind of beer hall bravado in Eckhof. If the military commanders Jellachic or Radetzky marched on the Austrian demonstrators instead of the Hungarians or Italians, wouldn't Eckhof quickly abandon the streets? And Rosenberg the Austrian? How much support would he give his Hungarian chief resident if Austrian Liberals turned against their Hungarian brethren. Would the First Clinic soon be much less of a sanctuary for Semmelweis?

He distrusted the depth of the students' commitment, just as he often distrusted the attachment of many surgeons to the well-being of their patients. Semmelweis suspected that he was surrounded by actors, and he remained cautious of everyone. This fearfulness only supplemented his reputation for arrogance. It also kept Doctor Semmelweis from trumpeting his astounding results in the battle against childbed fever. What folly it would be, Semmelweis thought, to present his theory about "cadaverous particles" now.

Semmelweis distrusted how much anyone would be willing to go to defend him. Yet he was touched by his students' faith in his innovations. The doctors, in turn, were more convinced than ever that Semmelweis had created an unprecedented medical earthquake. By the end of July 1848, the drastic drop in deaths from childbed fever in the First Clinic had lasted far more than a year. No longer could anyone proclaim, "The statistics this month mean nothing. The death rate always varies greatly."

Doctors were tallying their own numbers. Their combined statistics were always nearly identical to those of their chief resident. Since Semmelweis had cracked down severely on violations of his hand-washing decree, from February to the end of July, 1848, only eleven mothers in total had died from childbed fever. In July, 1848, there had been only one fatality.

He could almost hear his late friend, Professor Jakob Kolletschka, whispering in one ear, "Now is the time to make your move, Ignaz. Liberalism is on the rise. People will listen without prejudice." In his other ear, however, he heard the voice of another of his brothers, "European politics is like a great market that always advertises prices at ten percent of what they are elsewhere. And yet every day you go to that market, no matter how early in the morning, they are always sold out. Their shelves are forever empty. But, the people tell themselves, the prices are nevertheless miraculous."

"You must publish your results, Herr Doctor," many of his students urged him. But Semmelweis was afraid. As a Hungarian, he felt far more vulnerable to the storm outside the hospital than his non-Hungarian students.

Baron von Rokitansky did not want Semmelweis to publish, even though the other prominent Liberals at Vienna General Hospital were dispassionately following the results of the First Clinic experiment. The well-respected Professor von Hebra had already published two articles about Semmelweis's work by July, 1848. Semmelweis found his rare meetings with von Rokitansky bizarre. If his brother were to categorize the type of discourse between the chief resident and his famous teacher, Semmelweis had no doubt his brother would find it of the "non sequitur" variety.

Baron von Rokitansky summoned Semmelweis in late July. Semmelweis expected the usual curt, rapid-fire inquisition. He was not disappointed. Semmelweis supposed that the Baron felt it was his duty to interview Semmelweis every few months. The Baron began, "You are still applying the same number of leeches, Herr Doctor?"

"Yes, Herr Professor."

"It is the precise number Professor Klein has recommended?"

"Yes, Herr Professor."

"You are ensuring that there is adequate breeze through the clinic?"

"Yes, Herr Professor."

"You are giving the sick women frequent enemas and forcing them to vomit?"

"Yes, Herr Professor." Thank God there had been few ill women for over a year.

"You are still conducting autopsies?"

"Yes, Herr Professor."

"You remember that it was I who gave you permission to perform as many autopsies as you wish?"

"Yes, Herr Professor."

"You have conducted many autopsies, have you not?"

"I believe I have conducted far more autopsies personally than any other surgeon in the history of medicine, Herr Professor."

Semmelweis's former teacher winced. "You know that for many years I have taught that the knowledge we gain from forensic science will drive a revolution in medicine?"

"I was your dedicated student, Herr Professor. The whole sphere of European medicine has been your student."

"Everywhere they say that I have created a revolution in medicine. I have raised the reputation of medicine from its depths. I have based medicine on anatomy, on science. The days of medicine as a philosophy are gone. The time of superstitious practice is gone. I have seen that medicine is based on the human body. Do you think this is a good revolution, Herr Doctor Semmelweis?"

"Yes, Herr Professor."

"Do you believe doctors can know the human body without the knowledge that autopsies have given us?"

"No, Herr Professor."

"You have conducted a great many autopsies yourself?"

"Yes, Herr Professor."

"Your best friend, Professor Kolletschka, was a Professor of Forensic Science?"

"Yes, Herr Professor."

"You have kept your promise not to speak of 'cadaverous particles'?"

"Yes, Herr Professor."

"You no longer believe there is such a thing as cadaverous particles?"

"I do not know, Herr Professor," Semmelweis hedged. How could anyone not see the connection now between autopsies and the mysterious deaths of mothers?

It was not the reply that Professor von Rokitansky had wanted. His tone of voice changed. "Do you wish the disappearance of the Austrian Emperor?"

112

"No, Herr Professor."

"But you are Hungarian. Don't all Hungarians wish to be free of their king, the Austrian Emperor?"

"I don't think so, Herr Professor. There are as many opinions in Hungary as there are Hungarians."

"But your brothers work for Hungarian independence?"

"My brothers write to me only of the health of themselves and other family members."

"Hungary wants to abolish Jewish slavery. Lower Austria already has no Jewish slaves. The Emperor has never had any Jewish slaves. Your father was a Jewish merchant, was he not?

"I am Catholic, Herr Professor."

"You are not half-Jewish?"

"No, Herr Professor."

"So you say. You are dismissed, Semmelweis."

The distinguished Professor must have believed that he was being subtle with his sly questions. At the beginning of his residency, Semmelweis would have been thrilled for an audience before the esteemed Herr Baron von Rokitansky. Now the brief face-to-face interrogations by the Baron only frightened and depressed him. Liberals. Conservatives. A pox on both your houses, Semmelweis thought again as he left Professor von Rokitansky's office.

Yes, I did many post-mortems and then examined mothers about to give birth. Yes, we are all guilty, he would have told von Rokitansky if he had had more faith in his former teacher to discuss the situation reasonably. Science? A revolution in medicine? Yes, it still could be a new age for medicine, but von Rokitansky wanted to bury the connection between the frequency of autopsies and the previous epidemics of childbed fever. That would defeat the whole purpose of the revolution in medicine. In effect, to hide the truth might kill medicine itself.

Chapter Sixteen

The political tides turned again in August 1848. General Radetsky led soldiers on behalf of the Austrian Emperor and quickly defeated the Radicals in Vienna. The Austrian Emperor then returned to the city and appointed Conservatives as representatives. In other parts of the Empire the counterrevolution was also successful. Pest, the city near Semmelweis's hometown, was partially destroyed by the fighting.

Hungary, which had been the hope of the Viennese who opposed the Emperor, had had to fight many wars simultaneously. The new Hungarian government under Kossuth had established sweeping political and economic reforms in the spring of 1848, but had failed to satisfy Croats, Romanians, Serbs, and Slovaks. The Liberal Magyar government had limited the rights of Croatians and Romanians, and these Hungarian minorities saw no reason to substitute Austrian chains for Hungarian. The Kingdoms of Croatia and Slavonia declared themselves loyal to the Austrian Emperor, and appointed the Conservative Josip Jellacic as their leader. Jellacic had been removed from authority by a Liberal Hungarian government nominally loyal to the Austrian emperor. He set up a second Hungarian government, claiming fealty to the Emperor.

The Magyar Hungarians realized that they were at odds with all the minorities in the Kingdom of Hungary and, anticipating civil war, appealed to the Austrian Emperor for assistance. So that the Hungarian Magyars would be allowed to conscript an army, they promised the Emperor that they would send troops to northern Italy to support the Emperor in quelling an uprising there. The Emperor, however, ordered the Kingdom of Hungary not to raise an army. The leader of the Croats and Slovaks, Conservative Josip Jellacic, who claimed to be the rightful ruler of Hungary, then instituted military action against the Hungarian government without the blessing of the Austrian Emperor. At this point, Hungarian Radicals, who wanted complete independence from the Austrian Emperor, also moved against the Liberal Magyar government, which wanted to preserve a constitutional monarchy. The weakened Liberal government in Hungary was forced to make concessions to the Radicals.

The imperial court of Austria, after an attack on the non-Magyar Conservative military leader who had been given control of all Hungary armies, ordered the Hungarian government dissolved. The Conservative

Jellacic was appointed military leader over both Magyar Hungarians and the Hungarian minorities already in conflict with the Magyars. This finally precipitated war between Austria and Hungary

In Vienna in October, 1848, the Viennese Radicals, in support of their Hungarian allies, attacked soldiers on their way to reinforce Jellacic. The Radicals were quickly crushed. With order restored in Vienna, another 70,000 troops were sent to Hungary to crush the independence movement. In December the Hungarian government fled Pest.

The tide had turned against Liberalism. The promise of the Liberal spring of 1848 had become a resounding defeat for reform of the Austrian Empire. The struggle itself had weakened the Empire, had devastated Hungary. Moreover, it had strengthened nationalist tendencies in Europe.

How did this affect Doctor Ignaz Semmelweis and his crusade? In early 1849 it seemed as if the storms had passed over his corner of Vienna. The Conservative victory everywhere within the Austrian Empire seemed to have little effect on the day-to-day routine within the First Clinic and Vienna General Hospital, Medical and political discourse actually appeared at this time to be quite separate realms of reality. This impression was to later prove an illusion, but in the present there was great hope for the chief resident.

That was because in early 1849 Professor Joseph Skoda, one of the two doctors, along with Baron von Rokitansky, credited with founding the Modern Medical School of Vienna, came to see Semmelweis. Professor Skoda had quite a distinguished resume. He had served as a physician during a cholera outbreak in his native land, had been graduated from the University of Vienna Medical School, had been city physician of the poor in Vienna itself, and had been chief physician of the department of tuberculosis in Vienna General Hospital.

In 1846, because of Baron von Rokitansky's insistence, Skoda had been appointed professor of the medical clinic against the wishes of the entire medical faculty. Professor Skoda, a Czech Liberal, and Semmelweis the Hungarian thus had in common a history of surviving strong opposition. In addition the 45-year-old Skoda had been side-by-side with Semmelweis for 15 months, as the student apprenticed Skoda's methods. Professor Skoda, along with Baron von Rokitansky, had felt that Semmelweis was so promising he had also recommended Semmelweis for the position of chief resident.

"I always knew you would be successful," Professor Skoda told his prized student.

"This is indeed an honor, Herr Professor Skoda. I was quite happy to show you my results."

"I had no idea until I read of your innovation in your colleague's medical journal. He has published nothing more about your experiment since April of last year. I had to believe that since that time then the First Clinic must have retreated to the old situation, with death rates of 15% or more. I see now that I was mistaken. The death rate for all 1848 in the First Clinic was only 1.3%, exactly the same as the midwives' clinic."

"Yes, Herr Professor. I have kept very careful numbers. And if you talk to the doctors and midwives..."

"I have no need to do that, Ignaz. I trust you completely. I can see why those who are more distant from the wards themselves would look askance at your numbers, though. In the year before you arrived at the First Clinic more than ten times as many women died of childbed fever. You have nearly eradicated the disease. This is a miracle."

"Thank you, Herr Professor."

"I know your term as chief resident is expiring in a few weeks. The chief resident, of course, always receives an automatic two-year extension. Your predecessor, Herr Doctor Breit, was given that traditional honor and he is now a professor and the Chair of Obstetrics at the University of Tubingen, as you know. You have just as bright a future ahead of you after your residency, Ignaz."

"Thank you, Herr Professor. I am blessed to have been your student."

"Herr Professor von Rokitansky and I have both recommended that you should be reappointed for another two-year term as chief resident. Almost all of the medical faculty is also in favor of an extension. The few who have not spoken in your favor I suspect of extreme political bias and prejudice, Ignaz. No one can rationally deny what you have done. To try to erase or ignore your results would be insanity. You have begun one of the greatest advancements in medical history."

"Thank you, Herr Professor." Doctor Semmelweis was truly surprised by this praise and by the turn of events in his favor. He had become used to extreme criticism and mockery. He was shocked that Baron von Rokitansky was now favoring him. The Baron's attitude toward Semmelweis seemed to fluctuate according to the opinions around him. One of the founders of the revolution in medicine cared a great deal about the thoughts of his followers who hung on his every written and spoken word. That was a curious and dangerous situation.

"You may have saved all of us, Ignaz. You have revived the scientific revolution in medicine. When you arrived here in 1846 the poor women of Vienna called the days they were required to be examined by a doctor 'Death Days'. Our reputation was terrible, and yet we could not stop the tide of this disease that killed mothers. We were powerless."

"I myself could not sleep at night, Herr Professor."

"It seems so simple, the change that you have instituted. Yet you have revolutionized medicine, more so than Herr Professor von Rokitansky or I. The student now stands far taller than his teachers...."

"You give me too much credit. Herr Professor, please, it is not my intention at all to emerge from your shadow. I am quite grateful for my training. I am beholden to your teaching and your sponsorship."

"Do not protest, Ignaz. I do not accuse you of vanity and ambition. I only commend you for saving lives. I praise you for changing the entire current of ideas in medicine. Do not forget that I was the physician for the poor in this very city. I know the souls of these women that you have saved. I have compassion for them. Because of you no more can the people of Vienna claim that childbed fever is God's commandment that the poorer classes should not have children. You have not only changed medicine, Ignaz, but also religion and politics. Did you not realize this, Herr Professor?"

"Herr Professor, please...."

"Do not argue, Ignaz. I do not flatter you. I point you in the right direction. I urge you to have courage. Your students highly praise you, but they await your leadership. You have a great invention and do not speak nor write of it. The haughty English refer to you as either an idiot or a plagiarist of their idea. They tell everyone that somehow childbed disease traveled through the air from sick women to healthy women. And that they realized this true cause of childbed fever years before you came to Vienna General Hospital."

"Childbed fever is not caused by the exhalations of feverish women. That could not be possible."

"Because healthy women who have no contact with sick women still get childbed fever. Yes, you have made a scientific argument against the hubris of English medicine. Write and speak of this and save the mothers of England as you have rescued the mothers of Vienna. Because of you, Ignaz, Vienna is now again the center of medical knowledge for the world. You are the scientific revolution now. Tell the English they might as well blame vampire bats for childbed fever. Tell the English they should practice logical medicine as we do in Vienna. Tell the English to open their eyes and take the wax from their ears and to read and hear the truth. Tell them to try your innovations, and observe the results themselves."

"Herr Professor Klein would be disgusted with his chief resident if I did that."

"Who is Herr Professor Klein? Yes, he is the director of the clinic. Yes, he is your supervisor. And, yes, he is the one who will determine if you continue as chief resident for another two years. But he is not the young Herr Doctor Semmelweis, leader of a new revolution in medicine. If you are so worried about losing your position if you write articles and make speeches about your hand-washing bowls, then wait until your reappointment as chief resident. Continue to flatter Herr Professor Klein. Continue to trick him into believing that the drop in the deaths of mothers giving birth here is entirely due to him. Yes, Ignaz, I have guessed at your cleverness, but soon it will be the time to declare yourself. Soon you must emerge from your cocoon and save lives not just in Vienna, but all over the world.

"Your two-year term of reemployment as chief resident is automatic, Ignaz. Herr Professor Klein realizes this. He would not dare to dismiss you, not after what you have done for the reputation of doctors and Vienna General Hospital. Yes, doctors argue against you and try to get a piece of your invention. Surgeons are now horrified that the poor women of Vienna were always correct, that their 'autopsy hands' were what killed so many women, that 'Death Days' were, indeed, exactly that."

"I cannot ever forget, Herr Professor, that I myself performed more autopsies than any other doctor. I also encouraged my students to perform autopsies..."

"Just as you were encouraged to do by Herr Professor von Rokitansky and myself. We based our new revolution in medicine on the knowledge of anatomy."

"I blame no one more than myself. No ones hands have caused more death than mine. No ones hands were dirtier than mine when I went from an autopsy to a mother giving birth or to the examination of a new mother who had already given birth."

"You have upset your teacher, Herr Professor von Rokitansky. You pointed out that in 1823 when our scientific revolution began the death rate the previous year was less than 1%, that only 26 women had died of childbed fever in 1823. In 1823 when Herr Professor von Rokitansky began the scientific revolution in medicine and encouraged many more autopsies and extensive study of human anatomy, 214 women died in our clinic even though far fewer women gave birth here that year. The death rate for mothers was 7.5%.

"This is just sad truth. Ignaz. It is what happened. We gain nothing by burying the truth. You should continue. You should persevere in championing the truth."

"It is the sad truth for myself also, Herr Professor. I mean no insult to Herr Professor von Rokitansky or to yourself, Herr Professor. I am grateful for what you both have taught me."

"I take no offense, Ignaz. Of course not. I am happy for this new knowledge. Previously, I knew not what I had done, Ignaz. All doctors everywhere knew not what we had done. We were ignorant, and thought we were brilliant. Do not feel ashamed of the past, Ignaz. The far worst crime would be to continue our terrible practices in light of the new knowledge you have given us. Herr Professor von Rokitansky is deeply hurt. Of course he is. Doctors everywhere will be angry at first. How could they not be? You will be telling them that this new science that they have followed religiously for 26 years--26 years, Ignaz!--has always been the disease and not the cure. Of course they will be enraged. Everything they have believed--everything to which they have dedicated their lives--is now exposed as a deadly sham. No wonder you have been afraid to proclaim your miraculous discovery."

"What am I to say, Herr Professor? That some tiny particles on a scalpel entered the blood of Herr Professor Kolletschka and killed him, that a small cut on his finger was as deadly as if some madman had plunged the scalpel into his heart? I should tell the world that small bits from an autopsy are carried on a doctor's hands to the uterus of a mother and are as deadly as a thousand hammer blows to the head?"

"Yes. Yes. Say exactly this. Write exactly this. You have been Chosen, Ignaz. You cannot shirk your duty. Even if the whole world wants to crucify you for your truth. Show them your statistics. Show them your logic. Show them your science. Perhaps a few doctors will at first do everything in their power to deny your observations, even though it is obvious after all this time that your chlorinated-lime-and-water washing bowls save lives. A few doctors will not want to believe your dramatic decrease in the death rate for mothers. They will laugh at you because you have not found a cause that depends on an imbalance of humours or bad air or constipation as an explanation. They will call you a fool and a barber. They will not want to read your results nor hear your lectures. They will deny, deny, deny.

"But eventually they will all discover that you are right, Ignaz. They will slowly concede your truth, and the opposition to your discovery will gradually die out. Before your next two years as chief resident have expired, you will be a hero, Ignaz. You will have achieved, as Doctor von Hebra pointed out over a year ago, one of the greatest victories in medical history. Soon it will be time for you to conquer your fear and write of your simple innovation yourself, so that doctors everywhere can trust you and not wonder if your timidity is motivated by previous deceits."

"I am thrilled by your generosity, Herr Professor Skoda."

"I am not angry at you, Ignaz. I am quite proud of you. I will tell everyone everywhere that you were my student, that the student has achieved something far greater than that for which his teacher could ever aspire, that the student has taught Herr Professor Skoda and all of the Modern Medical School of Vienna a great lesson. Soon the revolution in scientific medicine begins anew with Herr Doctor Semmelweis's innovation and discovery as its starting point.

"A great new day for medicine begins soon, Herr Doctor Semmelweis."

Herr Professor Skoda left the office of Herr Doctor Semmelweis then. It had been a humble gesture for the prominent Professor to have visited Semmelweis's own office rather than having Semmelweis summoned. Doctor Semmelweis learned later that a colleague of his, Professor Ferdinand von Hebra, who had twice written of Semmelweis's dramatic successes in his well-respected medical journal, had appealed to Professor Skoda to ask his former student to begin explaining his method.

The visit by the medical pioneer for whom Doctor Semmelweis had been an assistant changed Semmelweis. He was now filled with new hope, confidence, and determination.

Chapter Seventeen

Professor Skoda's visit signaled a new beginning for Doctor Semmelweis's career and for the safety of mothers throughout Europe. Professor Skoda was perhaps second only to Professor Baron von Rokitansky in influence and in reputation. He had assured Semmelweis of another two years as the chief resident of the First Clinic.

"Of course," Professor Skoda had added. "Since Professor Klein is the director of the First Clinic, he must be the one to announce to you the two-year extension. It has always been a formality, however, and Professor Klein realizes this. In addition, there is the fact that Professor von Rokitansky, I, and nearly the entire medical faculty of Vienna General Hospital have strongly recommended you. Do you think that you can continue to attain the same results in the maternity clinics as you have for the last year and a half?"

"I am very confident that I can, Herr Professor."

"Then there will not be a doctor in the entire civilized world that can ignore the connection between the autopsies and childbed fevers. Soon you can feel secure enough to publish the results yourself, to demonstrate how the death rate rose when more autopsies were performed and the doctors went from the autopsy tables to the beds of the mothers and mothers-to-be. You can show what happened when you required doctors to wash their hands in chlorine water, how this nearly eliminated the childbed fevers. There is still some confusion about what you have achieved, Ignaz, and a great deal of resistance to the idea that doctors should have clean hands when they are examining their inferiors. You personally need to address these issues in a confident and clear way."

"I understand what you are saying, but you do not think I will still be mocked for blaming particles from the autopsied cadavers?"

"What difference does it make what you call the causative agent? What is critical is that you show the undeniable connection--the undeniable connection--between the autopsies and childbed fever. Nothing else matters. Your statistics, your success, the mothers who are now caring for their infants instead of resting far underground--this is the basis of the new scientific medicine. You are the pioneer and the teacher now, Ignaz--make the rest of the world understand your discovery."

Doctor Semmelweis followed the advice of his esteemed teacher. He became much bolder. He gathered his students and doctors and spoke to them of the death rate statistics, how the rate of deaths from childbed fever in 1823 rose to ten times the rate of the previous year because the scientific revolution in medicine had demanded a large increase in autopsies. The death of Professor Jakob Kolletschka from a scalpel cut on his finger during an autopsy had indicated some connection between the particles on the scalpel and childbed fever. The drastic reduction in deaths in the last year and a half from childbed fever simply by the introduction of hand-washing bowls in the clinic confirmed the connection."

Herr Doctor Miller rose during one of these informal lectures to shout out, "You lie, Semmelweis, you Hungarian pig. It is Professor Klein who is responsible for these results." But Miller was greeted only with derisive laughter. The doctors and students of the First Clinic knew what had caused the amazing change.

In January and February, 1849, there had been nearly 800 mothers admitted to the First Clinic, a large increase--the maternity clinic's reputation was at its zenith. There had been some carelessness. There were still doctors unconvinced that they could be the disease. Yet the death rate from childbed fever had remained low. Very few people now believed that there was no connection between autopsies that had been performed and deaths from childbed fever.

After Doctor Semmelweis had accompanied Professor Klein on rounds one morning in mid-March, the Professor informed Semmelweis that he needed to talk to him that afternoon about a matter of some importance. Doctor Semmelweis had become accustomed to the Professor's clipped attitude and revulsion toward wasting any but the most necessary words on Semmelweis, so he did not ask the purpose of the trip to the Professor's office. To visit the Director's office was an uncommon request. The Professor spent as little time as he could with his chief resident.

Semmelweis naturally assumed that Klein was to confirm his two-year extension as chief resident that Professors von Rokitansky and Skoda and the medical faculty of Vienna General Hospital had recommended.

In the afternoon, as he walked toward Professor Klein's office for his meeting, Doctor Semmelweis rehearsed the words he would use when he accepted his two-year employment extension. He must be humble, with no hint of emotion in his expression or voice. He must not seem like he was gloating. He needed to get along with Professor Klein, who would be his supervisor for another two years.

Soon he would publishing. Soon he, Doctor Semmelweis, could initiate a new era in the treatment of mothers everywhere.

Professor Klein, as usual, did not invite Semmelweis to be seated. He wasted no time nor words arriving at the point of the meeting. "Your commission expires on the 20th, Semmelweis. After that date you will no longer be employed at Vienna General Hospital."

"What?" Doctor Semmelweis gasped.

"Are you deaf, Semmelweis? You are no longer the chief resident of the maternity clinic. You are no longer employed at the First Clinic of Vienna General Hospital."

"That's impossible."

"No, Semmelweis, what you have been teaching is impossible. The situation you have created in the maternity clinic is impossible."

"I am recommended for an additional two years as chief resident by Herr Professor Rokitansky, by Herr Professor Skoda, by the medical faculty."

"I am the director of the clinic, not some foreign Liberals. I, and I alone, decide who is my chief resident."

"This is outrageous."

"No, Semmelweis, this is God's justice. Do you know how long I have waited for this moment? You were forced on me by those foreign Liberals, Skoda and von Rokitansky, and their friends. Now they must understand the political situation is not the same, and will never be the same. Now they will bow to the real rulers of medicine. By tonight, when they hear of how little I care about their recommendations, how little I have to fear their reputation and influence, they will realize that the brief era of Liberal ideas is now over. How long I have waited to bury all of you. How long I have wanted to banish the symbols of Liberal stupidity from my clinic. I have you to thank for giving me the means."

"Myself?"

"Your crazy ideas were the last straw for real doctors."

"When I arrived here, one of five mothers was dying of childbed fever. But recently in some months now we have no deaths at all."

"You fool. That's a coincidence. And, anyway, what do I care about peasant women and prostitutes? But you, Semmelweis, have told Austrian gentlemen their hands were too dirty to touch a whore. Who do you think you are? A Magyar and a whore may be equal, but neither should be dictating how an Austrian medical school graduate should act.

"We Austrian gentlemen hate you and Skoda and von Rokitansky and the rest of the foreign scum. How dare you. How dare you."

"How dare you, Professor? This is a clinic. Our job is to cure people and to save lives. Otherwise we are useless. Otherwise we are nothing. How dare you, Professor. I am doing what science revealed to me. I am treating the women under my care according to the real scientific methods. I have observed the technique that saves lives and I have used it. How can you call yourself a scientist? You are a fraud. How can you not care about that which saves these mothers? You would think that at the least you would care about your own reputation. You would think that at the minimum you would value the credibility of Vienna General Hospital."

"Two years ago did anyone care how many mothers died? Before you arrived here, Semmelweis, did anyone make a big noise about the difference in death rate between the First Clinic and the Second Clinic? It was nothing, a curiosity. Only you, Semmelweis, see something where better doctors see only air. We all thought that if we let you indulge yourself, you would eventually come to your senses. I gave you so many chances. I endured so much abuse and humiliation because of you, but thank God that nightmare is now finished. I was so sure that if I was patient and kind to you that you would come to your senses. But you haven't stopped. You just wouldn't stop.

"Your Liberal friends have written articles about your nonsense. It is an embarrassment to me. It's an embarrassment to the First Clinic, of which I am the director. It's an embarrassment to Vienna General Hospital and even to medicine itself. If you were here any longer, you would be The Death of Medicine."

"The Death of Medicine? I save lives. I save mothers."

"You embarrass us. You take some crazy idea and you imply that we are all murderers. Even your friend the Baron thinks so. What woman in Vienna would want to see a doctor now? The clown Semmelweis says we are all murderers. Don't go to a doctor, Semmelweis says. The doctor will kill you.

"There's actually people that believe you, Semmelweis. That's how terribly you poison the very air. I didn't realize until recently how powerful were the rumors you were spreading. I have been much too busy with other matters. The reputation of this clinic was sterling when you first arrived here. You and you alone have debased us. Everyone is afraid we will never recover from the lies you have told about the profession of medicine. You have thrown manure on the honor of us all.

"Now I am told you were deceiving me. I know about your trickery now. You were using your stupid wash bowls as a way to embarrass me and to replace me. You pretended to be my loyal servant. You secretly set yourself up as a hero, and I caught on to you too late. You are a clever conspirator, Semmelweis. Your deceit and ambition know no bounds. Everyone will know about your plot. Everyone will be sickened by the lies you have propagated. Every doctor in Europe is now labeled a murderer by your nonsense.

"Call me a murderer to my face like an honorable man. Address me with the same term you call me behind my back."

"I've never said anything like that. I've never called you a 'murderer' to anyone."

"You implied it. Don't deny it. Coward. Don't deny it. But you're too devious by far, Semmelweis. You never considered all the consequences of your trickery. You've damned your last supporters. Your friends, the Liberals von Rokitansky and Skoda and all the Liberals in their parade, you've condemned them as murderers, too."

"No. That's not true."

"Yes, Semmelweis. You are The Death of Medicine. Why should anyone want to see a doctor now? Doctors only want to kill women for their autopsies. Doctors are murderers. That is what you are trying to prove, Semmelweis. I know it. Professor von Rokitansky knows it. Everyone knows it. Where will you go now, Judas? The whole world will soon know of your plot."

"You misunderstand."

"No, I don't misunderstand you, Semmelweis. I suddenly see you for what you are. But let me tell you something. You have been too clever by far. I will tell everyone that you have proved Conservatives right. I will tell the world Semmelweis showed that the Conservatives were right. And it is true. We were correct. It is the Liberals who ordered the autopsies. It is the Liberals who wanted more and more autopsies. It is the Liberals who killed thousands of women. Go ahead, Semmelweis, lie about this. Deny it. You were the one that held a whip to the doctors and medical students. Perform more autopsies. Learn anatomy. Perform more autopsies.

"It was actually you who killed all those mothers. You forced students to perform the autopsies. You got their hands dirty, not me. You killed the mothers of Vienna, Semmelweis. Go ahead. Try and deny this fact."

"I do not."

"You have given Conservatives a great victory. Liberalism is death for women. This is what you have proven. This is what the world must soon say. Semmelweis proved it. Liberalism is death for women. For 26 years Liberals have been killing women with their experiments. You proved this, Semmelweis."

"So you will not continue the hand-washing bowls?"

"Did you hear me, Semmelweis? Have you heard a word I've said? No one believes your trickery, you deluded clown.

"Idiot. There are at least thirty causes for childbed fever. Even a medical student knows this fact. But you have accomplished one great feat, Semmelweis. No one will ever see Skoda and von Rokitansky and von Hebra as gods again. Even the people that believe your nonsense must condemn them all as murderers."

"So you will banish the clean hands that have saved so many women? What kind of a demon are you? You will let mothers die for the sake of your own reputation? You will only be a murderer. You will be a murderer if you tell the doctors they do not have to disinfect their hands between the time they finish an autopsy and when they examine the mothers in the clinic."

"I'm a murderer, Semmelweis? A murderer? You ungrateful piece of barbarian dirt. Get out. You will never work as a doctor again. You're finished, you piece of Magyar trash. I will tell the world of your plot to kill women for their corpses. You and von Rokitansky and Skoda. I will tell the world that God commanded me to save the mothers of the world from The Death of Medicine."

Doctor Semmelweis could think of no curse vile enough to hurl at the director of the First Clinic. He left quickly. He would never see Professor Klein again.

Doctor Semmelweis went to see Professor Skoda that evening. As Professor Klein had predicted, his teacher had been unmanned by Semmelweis's dismissal.

"I'm sorry, Ignaz. There's nothing I can do. What happened to you is unprecedented. A chief resident is automatically re-appointed for two years. I underestimated the depth of feeling against us." The Professor was extremely nervous, only one loud noise distant from trembling in fear. "We must wait. Perhaps in a few years the political situation will change again."

"Years?"

"There are times when a man must recede into the shadows. Sometimes we must retreat from wave after wave of ignorance. Sometimes it is better to be neither seen nor heard."

"But you told me the opposite. You told me to go forth boldly and to proclaim my successes. Wait? Sure, you can wait. You are still a doctor. You haven't been fired. You still have your position," Semmelweis said as a parting shot. You coward, he thought.

The visit to Professor Skoda's office had been an act of desperation. Skoda couldn't possibly override the decision by the director of the First Clinic. What could Semmelweis do now? Nothing. Where could Semmelweis turn to reverse the destruction of his career and reputation? Nowhere.

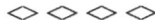

Professor Klein was right. Ignaz Semmelweis was never to work again as a doctor in Vienna. He did not immediately give up trying to find a new position. On the 20th of March he applied to become a private lecturer at the University of Vienna medical school. It would have been a humiliating downgrade for Semmelweis, but his former supervisor, Professor Klein, opposed his appointment. Semmelweis waited for more than a year and a half before giving up on Vienna. In May, 1851, disgusted with the medical establishment and their special interests, Doctor Semmelweis returned to Pest, Hungary. There he was appointed the director of the maternity clinic at Saint Rochus Hospital.

Doctor Semmelweis had been succeeded immediately at the Second Clinic by Doctor Braun, an obstetrician, an Austrian and a Conservative. He had been hand-picked by Professor Klein and held the chief resident position, assistant to Professor Klein, for more than four years. In March 1849, even though Semmelweis had nominally been at the clinic until the 20th, the death rate in the First Clinic doubled. It was to rise throughout the years of Doctor Braun's chief residency.

Doctor Braun wrote of 30 causes of childbed fever, and was very hostile to Semmelweis's idea of chlorine hand-washings. He did seem to throw a crumb to Semmelweis's successes, citing corpses as one of his 30 reasons for the fatal infections in mothers. However, Braun, like the English, blamed "miasms", evil thick vaporous exhalations from sick mothers, for spreading the disease. Braun is also famous for having a new ventilation system installed in the wards, claiming that it was bad air which had been a major cause of childbed fever. The deadly breath of sick mothers merely had to be blown away and the rate of childbed fever would decline.

The idea that there could be one single cause for childbed fever was everywhere regarded as ridiculous, despite the data that Semmelweis had accumulated. Doctor Semmelweis had taken a terrible fall from grace. He had no platform and no prestigious medical position by which he could use to demonstrate the effectiveness of hand-washing bowls.

As director of the maternity clinic at the small and backward Saint Rochus Hospital in Hungary he inherited the same situation, albeit on a smaller scale, as he had on his first day as chief resident of the First Clinic of Vienna General Hospital. Semmelweis was now back to square one.

In the ensuing years Doctor Carl Braun, Semmelweis's replacement in Vienna, was to receive honor after honor in his career. He received a knighthood, an ordinary professorship, and in 1856 he succeeded Professor Johann Klein as professor of obstetrics. For more than four years he was dean of the Vienna General Hospital medical faculty, and is remembered today as the man who made gynecology a discipline separate from other medical specialties. He eventually received an award reserved for only the most prominent professors.

Doctor Ignaz Semmelweis, in the meantime, set out his chlorine-and-water hand-washing bowls in the hell whose name had merely been changed from Vienna General Hospital to Saint Rochus Hospital. Semmelweis immediately achieved the same miracle results as he had in the First Clinic of Vienna General Hospital. From 1851-1855 Doctor Semmelweis lost only eight mothers from the 933 women who had given birth at Saint Rochus Hospital.

Childbed fever had been conquered by Doctor Semmelweis's innovation yet again.

Chapter Eighteen

Sometimes true life is much stranger than fiction. If this were a medical detective novel, then either the Liberals and Conservatives or both would have a change of heart (finally!) and sensible men would rise to power in the world of medicine. They would all advocate a doctor disinfecting his hands before examining a new mother or before assisting in the birth of a child. Some beneficent power would severely castigate the other doctors of Europe for their arrogance, greed, and stupidity, and strictly legislate hand-washing.

A good medical novel should end with the overwhelming majority of the population, of the professionals, and of the authorities all affirming the sanctity of human life, of common sense and observation, and of basic moral values over baser human selfishness.

That's not what happened. Acts III, IV, and V of Doctor Ignaz Semmelweis's adult life were lived exactly like Acts I and II, save for a change in location and the names of the bad actors. While Semmelweis believed he had presented startling evidence that could save the lives of women, everywhere in Europe doctors puffed themselves up and explained why Semmelweis was an idiot and why their theories about childbed fever were superior to those of everyone else.

It would be nice to be able to write that Doctor Ignaz Semmelweis, having achieved the same miracle in Hungary with his hand-washing bowls as he had in Vienna would now be proclaimed as a hero and genius.

That's not what happened. Semmelweis's innovation was not accepted by the other obstetricians even in Hungary. The most prominent of these preached that enemas were the best way to cure sick mothers, that childbed fever was due to a malfunctioning intestine. They would not listen to Semmelweis. Doctor Semmelweis had irritated the Hungarian doctors, probably because he had been safely in Austria during the terrible events of 1848 in the Kingdom of Hungary. When the leading professor of obstetrics at the University of Pest died in 1854, Semmelweis applied for the position. But so did Doctor Carl Braun, the man who had previously taken the chief residency position from Semmelweis in 1849 in Vienna. The majority of Hungarian doctors wanted Braun, even though Braun was Austrian, and did not speak Hungarian. In 1855 the authorities in Vienna overruled the Hungarian doctors' committee and appointed Semmelweis Professor of Obstetrics.

As he had in Vienna's First Clinic and in Hungary's Saint Rochus Hospital Doctor Semmelweis immediately set out his bowls of hand-wash in the University of Pest's maternity ward and explained their efficacy. Again he achieved miraculous results.

Doctor Semmelweis's chief resident, Doctor Josef Fleischer, printed an article proclaiming Semmelweis's near eradication of the fatal post-childbirth fevers. As the director of the Saint Rochus maternity clinic, Doctor Semmelweis had lost less than 1% of his patients, an astounding statistic in mid-nineteenth-century Europe. Yet the idea of chlorine hand-washings was still roundly mocked and Semmelweis was once again ridiculed for his ignorance.

The experts knew that no disease that had eluded revealing its mysteries for as long as childbed fever could possibly have only one cause. The notion that hand-washing bowls could prevent disease was ridiculous. The esteemed Professor Carl Braun, the doctor who had replaced Semmelweis in the First Clinic, had written the textbook explaining the thirty causes of childbed fever.

Doctor Semmelweis finally decided to explain himself. In 1858 he published "The Cause of Childbed Fever". In 1860 he published "The Difference in Opinion on the Subject of Childbed Fever between Myself and English Doctors", and finally in 1861 he published the much longer work which is considered his seminal work, "The Causes, Terms, and Prevention of Childbed Fever" (the approximate English equivalent of "Die Atiologie, der Begriff und die Prophylaxis des Kindbettfiebers").

Doctor Semmelweis had done what so many previously had asked of him. He had clearly written down his proof. He had revealed everything about his work, with neither guile nor shame. Now no one could deny the real cause of childbed fever. But in 1861, after the publication of his main work, most doctors in Europe again dismissed Semmelweis's simple innovation. Some were extremely rude in their condemnation of Semmelweis.

Many biographies of Semmelweis lose sympathy for the doctor after 1861. He was too loud. He was insulting. He was reckless. He was obsessed with the subject of childbed fever.

However, Doctor Semmelweis had tried every way possible to convince the medical community he could save lives. Now he no longer felt the need to be respectful and politic. What good had that attitude done? He sent scathing letters to the most eminent obstetricians and medical professors in

Europe (these messages were published as "Die Offener Brief", or "Public Letters") after his book was poorly received. He called the doctors the worst kind of names.

Some biographers of Semmelweis blame the doctor's rage in late 1861 and afterward as a large part of the reason that his innovations were not adopted. There were, allegedly, signs of severe mood swings, alcoholism, immoral behavior, and even Alzheimer's disease. Doctor Semmelweis had called some of the most revered physicians and medical professors in Europe "murderers" and "idiots". To the majority of learned men of science Doctor Semmelweis seemed bent on destroying their reputations. He literally was "The Death of Medicine".

By mid-1865 the medical community could no longer tolerate the behavior of the presumably alcoholic, demented, syphilitic Semmelweis. His friend, Doctor Ferdinand von Hebra, who was the first to champion Semmelweis's successes in his medical journal, was dispatched to put an end to the damage. He alleged had only the best interests of Semmelweis in mind and wanted to assist him. Doctor von Hebra was starting new maternity clinics, he told Semmelweis.

At last! Finally! The doctor who had first tried to tell the medical world that Semmelweis had made a profession-changing series of observations and connections now wanted Doctor Semmelweis to do for his new clinics what he had done for Vienna General Hospital's First Clinic, for Saint Rochus Hospital's maternity clinic, and for the University of Pest's maternity ward. Now Semmelweis had another opportunity to show the doctors of Europe that they had been unnecessarily killing women by the thousands.

But as Professor von Hebra was escorting Semmelweis on the tour of one of his new clinics, Doctor Semmelweis realized something was terribly wrong.

"This is not a maternity clinic!"

"No, Herr Doctor, it is an insane asylum."

And, as Doctor Semmelweis began to resist, as he tried to flee the trap, he was severely beaten. He soon developed an infection, and died a few weeks later of the same symptoms as his friend, Professor Jakob Kolletschka.

Doctor Ignaz Semmelweis, who in this twenty-first century is often referred to as "The savior of mothers", died of a form of what was then referred to as "childbed fever".

Epilogue

Doctor Ignaz Semmelweis was buried in Vienna on August 15th, 1865. Very few people in English-speaking countries have ever heard of him. He made the connection between autopsies and the death of mothers. He was the first to propose a simple single cause for childbed fever. He was an unstoppable force for medical science. He did not let his own prejudices nor those of his era deflect him from the undeniable conclusions of the data, even though it condemned him, his teachers, his colleagues, and all the doctors of Europe, England, and elsewhere as murderers of women.

Much is made of Louis Pasteur's "germ theory" as redemptive of Doctor Semmelweis's life work, and perhaps that is well and just, although it seems that calling that which jumped off the scalpel into Professor Kolletschka's blood a "germ" instead of a "cadaverous particle" isn't much of a theoretical advance. This is not to denigrate Pasteur's work in the least. I only point out the irony. Pasteur was, of course, French, and not Hungarian. Although Pasteur's experiments began during the time Doctor Semmelweis was working in Hungary, his theories only came to prominence long after the death of Doctor Semmelweis. What is critical is that Pasteur's ideas were not mangled by the political winds of the time.

During the years that obstetricians were trying to find a way to silence "The Death of Medicine" in the 1860s Pasteur was proving that fermentation was caused by the growth of mysterious micro-organisms, and not by some spontaneous generation. If Pasteur allowed no dust particles to reach his boiled broth, no fermentation occurred. Thus it was the dust particles that caused the change. If doctors washed particles from their hands using Doctor Semmelweis's bowls of lime and water, no mothers died of disease. Thus it was the particles that caused the disease. Louis Pasteur is remembered gratefully. The virtually unknown Doctor Ignaz Semmelweis to this day still must contend with charges of alcoholism, dementia, and lewd and syphilitic behavior that may or may not be true. Moreover, these unprovable speculations are irrelevant to the example of dedication he bequeathed to medicine and humanity.

www.ingramcontent.com/pod-product-compliance
Lightning Source LLC
Chambersburg PA
CBHW051540170526
45165CB00002B/807